EYE AND VISION RESEARCH DEVELOPMENTS

RECENT ADVANCES IN OPHTHALMOLOGY RESEARCH

Eye and Vision Research Developments

Additional books in this series can be found on Nova's website under the Series tab.

Additional e-books in this series can be found on Nova's website under the e-book tab.

EYE AND VISION RESEARCH DEVELOPMENTS

RECENT ADVANCES IN OPHTHALMOLOGY RESEARCH

GALINA DIMITROVA
EDITOR

NOVA BIOMEDICAL

New York

For permission to use material from this book please contact us:
Telephone 631-231-7269; Fax 631-231-8175
Web Site: http://www.novapublishers.com

Additional color graphics may be available in the e-book version of this book.

Library of Congress Cataloging-in-Publication Data

ISBN: 978-1-62808-021-6

Library of Congress Control Number: 2013939758

Published by Nova Science Publishers, Inc. † New York

Contents

Preface

This book is a collection of relevant topics dealing with recent advances in ophthalmology research. The selected review studies present novel investigation and prospects in ophthalmology concerning ocular stem cells, neurodegeneration, immunology, angiogenesis treatment, and the research of ocular blood flow. All of the authors of this collection are experts in the topics they present.

In Chapter 1, Stewart discusses treatment options for conditions considered major causes of blindness in industrialized countries (age-related macular degeneration, diabetic retinopathy, and retinal vein occlusions). These diseases are associated with upregulation of vasoproliferative factors, such as VEGF-A, VEGF-B, and placental growth factor. VEGF has been recognized as a critical growth factor for both physiologic and pathologic angiogenesis. The author reviews the pharmacokinetic behaviors of the available anti-VEGF drugs and discusses these characteristics in conjunction with mathematical modeling to explain the results seen in clinical trials and to predict the responses in still untested circumstances.

Dimitrova and Kato (Chapter 2) present the methods of ocular blood flow research. The investigation of ocular circulation is an important segment in the research of ophthalmic physiology and pathophysiology. The ocular vascular system is quite complex and the methods of ocular blood flow measurement investigate different aspects of blood flow in specific vascular beds. The authors discuss the specifics of the ocular vascular system and make an overview of the currently used methods of ocular blood flow. Novel applications and technology in ocular circulatory research are addressed.

In Chapter 3, Park and Ou correlate the pathogenetic mechanisms of two relevant neurodegenerative diseases – glaucoma and Alzheimer's disease

(AD). Glaucoma is among the leading causes of blindness in the world today, while AD is a highly debilitating disease causing a major social and economic impact to our society. Glaucoma and AD are thought to share, at least in part, some commonalities, as both are age-related neurodegenerative diseases. The authors refer to several studies that report higher prevalence of glaucoma in patients with AD, than in control subjects, which suggests a link between the two conditions. In their review, the authors explore this possible link in the context of the axon, dendrite, and synapse. They report a growing body of evidence supporting the idea of compartmentalized degeneration of retinal ganglion cells in glaucoma. Discovering earlier disease markers and novel therapeutic targets at multiple subcellular compartments will likely be necessary to adequately subdue disease progression in glaucoma.

Both innate and adaptive immunity take part in the defensive systems of the ocular surface. Rania et al. (Chapter 4) discuss the innate immunity mechanisms that are involved in dry eye syndrome, an inflammatory condition of the ocular surface derived by tear hyperosmolarity consequent to either increased tear evaporation or aqueous deficiency. The authors present the promoters for innate immunity of the ocular surface and discuss them in context of the dry eye syndrome. The comprehension of the molecular basis of dry eye disease may help identify the biomarkers that could help the differentiation between patients and normals, but also from other diseases with overlapping characteristics, such as seasonal allergic conjunctivitis.

Dhamodaran et al. (Chapter 5) discuss novel investigation about using stem cells in ophthalmology. The potentials and characteristics of these cells categorize them under a different group from other cell types of the body. Stem cells are unspecialized cells harboring proliferative and differentiative properties to become tissue or organ specific cells. Among all the branches of health sciences, ophthalmology may be the first to get the benefits of stem cell treatment. The eye, being an immune privileged organ, fulfills all the necessary criteria for stem cell treatment and research. The most wide and successful use of adult stem cells in treatment is limbal epithelial cell transplantation for removing corneal scar or involving patients with limbal stem cell deficiency. The use of stem/progenitor cells for remedy or prevention of ocular disease progression implies a great expectation. This chapter addresses different aspects of stem cells use in treating ocular diseases, including the ongoing research efforts and the future prospects.

This collection is intended for ophthalmologists, as well as for medical doctors from other specialties and medical students who have interest in the field of ophthalmology. The information presented here has both scientific and clinical relevance for the reader. This book has been conceived and prepared with expectation that it would add new insights and inspiration for the clinicians and researchers who deal with patients suffering from ophthalmic diseases.

In: Recent Advances in Ophthalmology Research ISBN: 978-1-62808-021-6
Editor: Galina Dimitrova

Chapter 1

The Pharmacological Behavior of Anti-VEGF Drugs: Implications for the Treatment of Age-Related Macular Degeneration

Michael W. Stewart[*]
Department of Ophthalmology, Mayo Clinic, Florida, US

Abstract

The importance of a soluble vascular growth factor to support the angiogenesis that is essential for both tumor growth and ocular neovascularization had been postulated for decades. The search for this factor led to the discovery of vascular endothelial growth factor (VEGF) in 1989, followed by 2 decades of intense and productive research. VEGF has subsequently been recognized as a critical growth factor for both physiologic and pathologic angiogenesis. VEGF expression results in migration and proliferation of vascular endothelial cells, breakdown of tight junctions, dissolution of the intercellular matrix, vascular dilation and attraction of endothelial cell progenitors and monocytes.

Major causes of blindness in industrialized countries (age-related macular degeneration, diabetic retinopathy and retinal vein occlusions) are associated with upregulation of VEGF-A, VEGF-B and placental

[*] E-mail: stewart.michael@mayo.edu.

growth factor. Since pre-clinical studies demonstrated that blocking the actions of VEGF prevents the growth of experimental choroidal neovascularization (CNVM), four drugs (pegaptanib, bevacizumab, ranibizumab and aflibercept) that prevent VEGF from binding to its cognate receptors have been developed. Pivotal phase 3 trials showed that intravitreal injections of these drugs every 4 to 8 weeks prevent moderate loss of vision in most patients and significantly improve vision in a significant number. However, there exist differences in the peak effects and durations of action between these. As a result, some patients fail to respond to standard therapeutic regimens. When confronted with these patients, surgeons must consider changing one of the following: the drug, the administered dose, or the frequency of injections. Mathematical modeling based on pharmacokinetic data has been able to explain many of the observed clinical findings and successfully predict the results of untested alternative therapeutic strategies. This chapter will review the pharmacokinetic behaviors of the available anti-VEGF drugs and use these characteristics in conjunction with mathematical modeling to explain the results seen in clinical trials and to predict the responses in, as yet, untested circumstances.

Keywords: Aflibercept, bevacizumab, pegaptanib, pharmacokinetics, ranibizumab, vascular endothelial growth factor, VEGF

Introduction

The development and widespread use of drugs that prevent the actions of vascular endothelial growth factor (VEGF) has improved survival in patients with advanced solid tumors [46,91] and completely revolutionized the treatment of chorioretinal vascular diseases [7,9,12,77,88]. Since the leading causes of blindness in industrialized countries are VEGF-driven processes [1,58], the use of these drugs by ophthalmologists has risen dramatically since they became available. Well-designed trials have demonstrated that both regular and as-needed (with regular evaluations) intravitreal injections prevent vision loss in the overwhelming majority of patients and improved vision in a large percentage [5,9,10,13,61,77,90].

Not all patients, however, are treated according to trial protocols. Many patients do not require monthly (or bimonthly) intravitreal injections so physicians attempt to lengthen the inter-treatment intervals [22,23,38,47]. On the other hand some patients respond poorly to monthly injections and require the use of other treatment strategies [84].

The purpose of this chapter is to discuss important aspects of VEGF biochemistry, the chemical properties and pharmacokinetic characteristics of the available anti-VEGF drugs, and the pharmacokinetic rationale for treatment strategies that can be employed to treat special situations.

VEGF

The path to VEGF discovery included contributions from clinical researchers and basic scientists with diverse backgrounds. Michaelson (1948) first proposed the existence of a soluble vasoproliferative factor "X" that caused neovascular growth in conditions such as diabetic retinopathy [64]. Folkman (1971) suggested that solid tumor growth depended on the secretion of an angiogenic factor [28]. Senger (1983) identified a protein called "vascular permeability factor" but the technology available at the time prevented complete sequencing of the molecule [79]. Finally, two independent groups (1989) isolated identical angiogenic proteins and further testing showed that these were identical to the previously identified vascular permeability factor [15,27].

The newly discovered molecule, vascular endothelial growth factor, is actually several molecules that segregate into 6 families: VEGF-A, VEGF-B, VEGF-C, VEGF-D, VEGF-E and placental growth factor [25,66]. Native VEGF exists as a mixture of homodimers with an average molecular weight of 45 kDa [44]. The biological roles of the different families are not completely understood but VEGF-A appears to be critical for the angiogenesis and hyperpermeability steps necessary to support tumor growth [25] and cause the vascular abnormalities seen in ophthalmic chorioretinal vascular diseases [59]. VEGF-A is made up of 6 major isoforms ($VEGF_{121}$, $VEGF_{145}$, $VEGF_{165}$, $VEGF_{183}$, $VEFF_{189}$ and $VEGF_{206}$) and at least 8 minor isoforms [44,89]. $VEGF_{165}$, the predominant isoform, is responsible for most VEGF-related angiogenic processes [47,62].

Each $VEGF_{165}$ molecule contains 2 binding sites: the receptor binding site resides within amino acids 81 through 92, and the heparin binding site resides within amino acids 110 through 165 [52]. Therefore, all VEGF-A isoforms including the cleaved product $VEGF_{110}$, can bind to VEGF receptors. However, only isoforms with 165 amino acids or more contain the heparin binding site which allows VEGF to interact with neuropilins, become sequestered within the intercellular matrix, or bind to cell membranes [73].

Shorter isoforms of VEGF-A (i.e. those with 145 amino acids or fewer) are freely diffusible. On the other hand, isoforms longer than 165 are highly basic and are sequestered within the intercellular matrix - $VEGF_{165}$ has intermediate solubility characteristics since 50% to 70% of it is matrix bound - thereby creating a reservoir of potentially active VEGF [73]. When tissues become ischemic or are subjected to inflammation, matrix metalloproteinase-9 dissolves the extracellular matrix thereby allowing plasmin to cleave the sequestered isoforms into biologically active, soluble $VEGF_{110}$ [45,73].

Diffusible VEGF dimers bind to the exodomains of three trans-membrane receptors: VEGFR1(flt-1), VEGFR2 (flk-1) and VEGFR3 (flk-4). Each receptor contains VEGF binding sequences within the extracellular segments, a trans-membrane segment, and an intracellular portion with tyrosine kinase moieties [16,86]. When VEGF binds to the extracellular domain, the receptors dimerize, the intraocular tyrosine kinase moieties become phosphorylated, and several biochemical signaling pathways become activated, thereby causing physiologic effects downstream [11,21,37,85]. Co-receptors, called neuropilins, bind to the heparin binding sequences of $VEGF_{165}$ and favorably present the dimer to the extracellular receptor sequences to amplify the resultant signal strength by up to 10-fold [30].

The physiologic response caused by VEGF is determined by both the particular family and isoform of VEGF and the activated receptor. VEGF-B [51] and placental growth factor (PlGF) [71] bind only to VEGFR1 whereas VEGF-A binds to both VEGFR1 and VEGFR2 [26]. VEGFR1 appears to play a minor role in the development of most angiogenesis but it appears to serve in other capacities.

For example, VEGFR1 activation by VEGF-B regulates coronary artery development [56], whereas activation by VEGF-A results in monocyte chemotaxis [19]. Some investigators believe that VEGFR1 binding of PlGF, displaces VEGF-A and allows it to bind to VEGFR2 [73]. By this mechanism VEGFR1 promotes angiogenesis by acting as a "dummy" receptor. Since recent evidence shows that both placental growth factor [76] and VEGF-B [95] are associated with choroidal neovascularization, direct VEGFR1 stimulation may result in angiogenesis.

Most of the angiogenic processes associated with tumor growth and ocular angiogenesis, however, result from VEGF-A binding to VEGFR2. Receptor activation phosphorylates intraocular enzymes that upregulate RAF/MEK/ERK, phosphotidylinositol 3-kinase, and MAPK pathways [11,21,37,85]. These lead to vascular endothelial cell proliferation, swelling and migration, breakdown of the blood-retinal barrier, dissolution of the intercellular matrix, and improved cell survival [26,92]. The nature and strength of the physiologic response depends upon the concentration of VEGF, with lower concentrations resulting in breakdown of the blood-retinal barrier and higher concentrations leading to angiogenesis in the form of retinal or choroidal neovascularization [52].

Drug Development

Angiogenesis may be stimulated by several growth factors (acidic and basic fibroblastic growth factors, insulin-like growth factor, transforming growth factors α and β, platelet derived growth factor, angiopoietins 1 and 2, VEGF), inflammatory cytokines (interleukin-8) and metabolic conditions (hypoxia) [6,29,93]. For most ocular neovascular conditions (e.g. age-related macular degeneration, proliferative diabetic retinopathy and retinal vein occlusions) hypoxia is a critical driver [66]. Low oxygen concentrations stabilize hypoxia inducible factor-1α (HIF-1α) by preventing its hydroxylation by propyl hydroxylases.

The stabilized HIF-1α is unable to bind with the Von-Hippel factor and instead it dimerizes with HIF-1β, thereby avoiding ubiquination and degradation within proteosomes. The HIF dimer then binds to the promoter region of the VEGF gene and initiates VEGF mRNA synthesis [54,60]. VEGF diffuses through ocular tissues into the vitreous creating higher concentrations adjacent to ischemic retina and lower concentrations in the more distant anterior and central vitreous. When tissue concentrations of VEGF are sufficient to initiate new blood vessel development, growth occurs in the direction of the highest VEGF concentrations.

Since VEGF is both sufficient and necessary for angiogenesis, VEGF biochemistry has been intensively studied and well characterized. Not surprisingly, limiting tumor growth and reversing vision loss due to chorioretinal vascular disorders by limiting the effects of VEGF on vascular endothelial cells became an early strategy employed by drug developers. Several development strategies have been employed, some of which have led to the development and regulatory approval of drugs with anti-VEGF actions. Tyrosine kinase inhibitors, small molecules that can be administered orally, easily cross cell membranes, inhibit the phosphorylation of intraocular moieties, and prevent the activation of downstream stimulatory biochemical pathways. Tyrosine kinase inhibitors are capable of inhibiting leakage from choroidal neovascular membranes, but because of possible adverse events due to systemic VEGF suppression, they have been used on only a few patients [17]. Antibodies to VEGFR2 have been used in experimental models but have not been developed for human use.

Drug development for human use has focused on preventing the activation of VEGF receptors by binding soluble VEGF (Figure 1). Three major strategies have been pursued: aptamer technology, antibody-based drugs, and fusion proteins that contain native VEGF-receptor sequences. The first ophthalmic anti-VEGF drug, pegaptanib (Macugen®, Eyetech, Palm Beach Gardens, FL), is a pegylated aptamer that binds to the heparin-binding domain of longer VEGF isoforms [67]. Since $VEGF_{189}$ and $VEGF_{206}$ are nearly entirely bound to the intercellular matrix and cell membranes, pegaptanib exerts its inhibitory effects by binding exclusively to diffusable $VEGF_{165}$. Receptor binding is prevented because the drug's size interferes with VEGF-VEGFR2 interaction. Unfortunately, naturally occurring, shorter VEGF isoforms such as $VEGF_{145}$ and $VEGF_{121}$, and the cleavage product $VEGF_{110}$ are unaffected by pegaptanib [47].

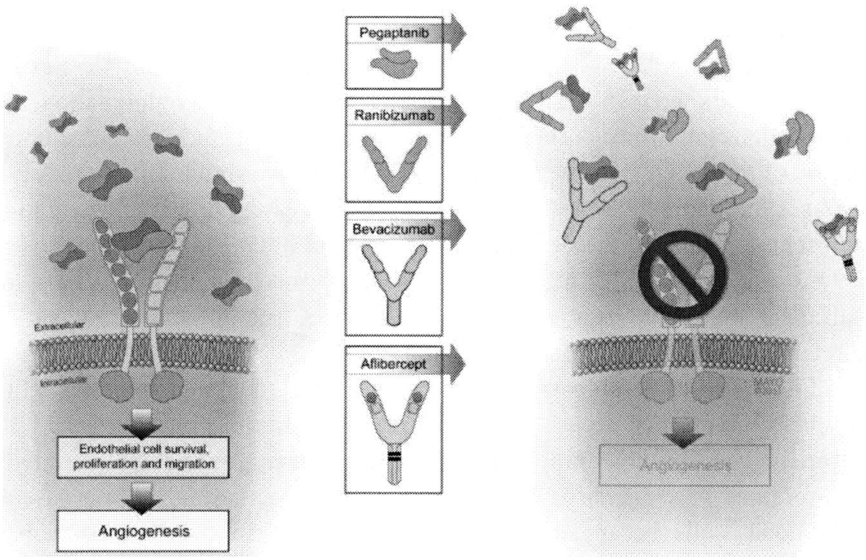

Figure 1. The left panel shows how VEGF dimers (green figures) interact with the extracellular binding domains of the trans-membrane VEGF receptor molecules, resulting in receptor dimerization, endothelial cell activation and ultimately, angiogenesis. The right panel shows how the 4 anti-VEGF drugs (pegaptanib, bevacizumab, ranibizumab, aflibercept) bind VEGF, thereby preventing its interaction with the receptors.

The most commonly employed inhibition strategy involves binding soluble VEGF before it can activate its cognate receptors. Bevacizumab, a humanized antibody that binds all isoforms of VEGF-A, was the first antibody-based, anti-VEGF drug to gain regulatory approval. Bevacizumab contains 2 VEGF binding sites, thereby binding VEGF in 1:1 and 1:2 ratios [48]. Since VEGF is a dimer, large macromolecular aggregates called "daisy chains" can be formed. The significance of these aggregates is not fully known but they may explain the higher incidence of anti-VEGF induced glaucoma that has been reported with bevacizumab [35].

The intraocular pharmacokinetic properties of bevacizumab have been well studied in both animal models and humans. Following the intravitreal injection of bevacizumab, its concentration decreases according to a first order kinetic model. The half-life of bevacizumab in rabbit eyes is 4.2 to 4.3 days, as measured by PET-CT (radioactive-labeled bevacizumab) [14] and by intravitreal sampling and quantification with ELISA assays [4]. After injection into the vitreous, bevacizumab reaches the subretinal space in rabbits within 2 hours [18] and the RPE and choroid of monkeys within 24 hours [40]. Peak bevacizumab concentrations within the rabbit retina (93,990 ng/gm) exceed those within the vitreous (59,730 ng/gm), suggesting the sequestration and concentration of bevacizumab [70]. Bevacizumab exits the eye through both the anterior chamber and the choroidal circulation [4] without undergoing degradation within the eye. The intraocular half-life of bevacizumab in monkey eyes has not been measured but that of herceptin (a comparable full-length antibody) is 5.6 days [65].

The intraocular half-life of bevacizumab in humans ranges from 6.9 days to 9.8 days (average of 8.25 days) [53,63,96]. Meyer et al [63] determined that doubling the intravitreal dose from 1.5 mg to 3 mg did not prolong the half-life, but that it extended the treatment duration by one half-life.

Bevacizumab has a long half-life (21 days) in the systemic circulation because the molecule's Fc fragment minimizes glomerular filtration and renal excretion [36]. Following intraocular injections into one eye, low levels of bevacizumab have been detected in the contralateral eyes of rabbits [4], and regression of proliferative diabetic retinopathy has been observed in the contralateral eye in humans [3]. These observations suggest that low, but perhaps therapeutic, bevacizumab concentrations may enter non-injected eyes from the systemic circulation. Monthly intravitreal bevacizumab injections have been shown to decrease systemic VEGF levels [13].

After intravitreal injections of ranibizumab into rabbit eyes, the intraocular half-lives range from 2.1 to 3 days by ELISA [4,34] and PET-CT (after radioactive iodine labeling) [14]. Ranibizumab has a half-life of 2.6 to 3.2 days in monkey eyes [33,65] and though human experimental data is not available, estimates of its intraocular half-life range from 4.79 days (adapted mathematical model) [81] to 9 days (human population kinetics study) [39]. Ranibizumab penetrates the retina and choroid quickly and reaches peak concentrations that are 1/3 and 1/6 those measured within the vitreous [33]. Since ranibizumab is rapidly excreted by the kidneys, its systemic half-life is quite short (3 hours in rabbits) [32]. As a consequence, intravitreal ranibizumab therapy does not result in a sustained decrease in serum VEGF levels [13] and ranibizumab has not been detected in fellow eyes [4].

Available pharmacokinetic data for aflibercept is considerably more limited. Its intraocular half-life in rabbits is 4.7 days [31] and though human data does not exist, the half-life of aflibercept has been estimated to be 7.1 days [81]. Aflibercept binds VEGF quickly within the systemic circulation (half-life of unbound aflibercept is 1 to 3 days) and is cleared (probably by proteolysis) slowly after binding VEGF (half-life of VEGF-bound aflibercept is 18 days) [87]. This long half-life is probably due to the large Fc segment which prevents glomerular filtration. Patients with exudative AMD who were treated with intravenous aflibercept (0.3 mg/kg and 1 mg/kg) achieved modest gains in vision but did not have detectable aflibercept in the serum at 1 month; only patients receiving 3 mg/kg had measurable serum levels, but 2 of these 5 patients suffered from dose-limiting toxicity [69]. Therefore, effective treatment of CNVM could not be safely given with monthly intravenous injections. For this reason all subsequent ophthalmic trials with aflibercept were performed with intravitreous injections.

Drug Actions

After the intravitreal injection of an anti-VEGF drug, binding with VEGF occurs rapidly:

Drug + VEGF = Drug-VEGF

Though this binding is reversible, the very small dissociation constants possessed by each of the available drugs means that binding occurs rapidly with the majority of available VEGF. After intraocular injections of anti-VEGF drugs, their intraocular concentrations decrease in an exponential manner. This results in a slow increase in the concentration of unbound VEGF until it reaches a concentration sufficient to reactivate the hyperpermeability and proliferative processes. At all times, the equilibrium between free drug, bound VEGF, and unbound VEGF is maintained according to the following equation:

$$\text{Drug} + \text{VEGF} \overset{K_d}{\leftrightarrow} \text{Drug} + \text{VEGF}$$

where the dissociation constant (K_d) is represented by

$$K_d = [\text{Drug}]\,[\text{VEGF}] \,/\, [\text{Drug-VEGF}]$$

and with algebraic manipulation

$$[\text{Drug}] \,/\, K_d = [\text{Drug-VEGF}] \,/\, [\text{VEGF}]$$

The term on the right side of the equation ([Drug-VEGF]/[VEGF]) represents the proportion of VEGF which is bound by the drug. Though the value of this term cannot be easily determined, the term on the left side of the equation ([Drug]/K_d) can be estimated for each drug from known parameters (dissociation constants, injected drug volumes and intravitreal half-lives).

Similar molar amounts of each of the 3 commonly used anti-VEGF drugs are injected into eyes. Commonly injected volumes (0.05 ml) of each commercial product produce the following relative initial intravitreal molar concentrations: ranibizumab - 1, bevacizumab – 0.8, and aflibercept – 1.67.

The dissociation constant (K_d) measures the drug's proclivity to separate from VEGF (the reverse of binding), so a lower dissociation constant means a "stickier" molecule with a higher binding affinity for VEGF. Dissociation constants for each drug have been studied by numerous investigators and vary from study to study. Dissociation constants for bevacizumab vary between 58 pM and 1.1 nM [72,75]; for ranibizumab they vary from 46 pM to 192 pM [24,72], whereas aflibercept's values fall within a much narrower range, from 0.5 pM to 1.0 pM [43,72]. Furthermore, aflibercept binds both PlGF-2 (K_d = 45 pM) and VEGF-B with high affinity [43].

The ability of these drugs to prevent vascular endothelial cell activation (proliferation and migration) in cell cultures has also been studied. Ranibizumab is between 5x and 20x as effective as bevacizumab at preventing endothelial cell activation [24]. A study comparing ranibizumab, bevacizumab and a VEGF Trap construct (similar to aflibercept) showed that ranibizumab and the VEGF Trap were equally effective at preventing endothelial cell proliferation and migration, and both were 11x as effective as bevacizumab [94]. A similar study by different researchers showed that aflibercept was 27x to 129x as effective as bevacizumab and ranibizumab at decreasing calcium mobilization and 10x to 100x as effective at decreasing endothelial cell proliferation [72]. The reason for the striking differences between the results of the two studies is not clear, but one of the authors attributed it to the different concentrations of VEGF used (1000-fold higher in the first study) [72].

Early dose-escalating trials for ranibizumab and aflibercept aimed to establish the efficacy and safety of different doses of each drug. Pre-clinical studies with ranibizumab suggested that the clinical effect would last for one month following an intravitreal injection [33] and the phase 1 and 2 trials supported this conclusion [41,82]. Therefore, clinical efficacy in phase 3 trials was generally measured by the drug's ability to prevent loss of vision, by the number of letters gained, and by the amount of thinning of the macula after patients received monthly injections. In the dose escalation trials, higher doses generally produced greater clinical effects [41,82]. Ranibizumab appeared to be effective at a dose of 0.5 mg and since the 2 mg preparation appeared highly viscous, the phase 3 trials featured only the 0.3 mg and 0.5 mg doses [9,77]. Early data suggested that higher doses of anti-VEGF drugs produced greater peak effects than lower doses [8,42,68]. However, subsequent observations suggest that most doses give comparable clinical effects if the inter-injection intervals are appropriately adjusted.

Even relatively small amounts of anti-VEGF drugs (certainly much smaller than those given intravitreally in early trials) bind the overwhelming majority of free VEGF and temporarily halt angiogenesis. However, as the intraocular concentration of a drug decreases with time, the biological effects achieved with small drug doses wear off much quicker than those with larger doses. So when patients are evaluated at monthly intervals the peak effects from lower doses are probably not seen because the clinical effect has since worn off.

The phase 3 MARINA [77] (Minimally Classic/Occult Trial of the Anti-VEGF Antibody Ranibizumab in the Treatment of Neovascular Age-Related Macular Degeneration Study) and ANCHOR [9] (Anti-VEGF antibody for the Treatment of Predominantly Classic Choroidal Neovascularization in Age-Related Macular Degeneration Study) trials compared both 0.3 mg and 0.5 mg doses of ranibizumab to observation (MARINA) and photodynamic therapy (ANCHOR). With monthly administration, the 0.5 mg dose was found to produce superior gains in vision compared to the 0.3 mg dose (MARINA: +7.2 letters vs. +6.5 letters; ANCHOR: +11.3 letters vs. +8.5 letters). The 2 mg dose of ranibizumab was subsequently compared to 0.5 mg (with monthly and PRN regimens) in the HARBOR trial [10]. The gains in vision at one year were comparable in both the monthly arms (0.5 mg: +10.1 letters; 2 mg: +9.2 letters) and the PRN arms (0.5 mg: +8.2 letters; 2 mg: +8.6 letters). In the PRN arms, patients receiving 0.5 mg required 7.7 injections whereas patients receiving 2 mg required only 6.9 injections.

The phase 1 trial with aflibercept featured escalating doses from 0.05 mg to 4 mg. At 6 weeks patients receiving single injections of 2 mg and 4 mg experienced superior thinning of the macula (-216 μm) compared to those receiving 0.05 mg to 0.5 mg (+9 μm) [68]. As a result, during the first 16 weeks of the phase 2 study, doses of 0.5 mg, 2 mg and 4 mg were administered quarterly and doses of 0.5 mg and 2 mg were administered monthly. During the first phase of the study, patients receiving monthly injections experienced greater thinning of the macula than those dosed quarterly [8].

The phase 3 VIEW 1 and 2 trials featured 4 treatment arms: monthly aflibercept 0.5 mg, monthly aflibercept 2 mg, every 8 weeks aflibercept 2 mg, and monthly ranibizumab. All aflibercept arms achieved the primary endpoint: non-inferiority compared to ranibizumab for preventing 15 letter loss of vision (aflibercept: 95% to 96%; ranibizumab: 94%). Furthermore, all aflibercept arms produced comparable gains in vision (+6.9 letters to +10.9 letters) compared to ranibizumab (+8.1 letters and +9.4 letters). The only exception was the aflibercept 2 mg every 4 week arm in the VIEW 1 in which patients gained +10.9 letters compared to +8.1 letters in the ranibizumab group ($p = 0.001$). Interestingly, the 2 doses of monthly aflibercept produced comparable gains in vision (aflibercept 0.5 mg: +6.9 letters and +9.7 letters; aflibercept 2 mg: +10.9 letters and 7.6 letters) [5].

These data suggest that further increasing the dose of a drug that improves vision at one month does not result in additional gains in vision. Increasing the dose, however, appears to prolong the duration of action. Patients receiving the 2 mg dose of ranibizumab in the HARBOR trial [10] required fewer injections than those receiving the 0.5 mg dose (6.9 vs. 7.7), suggesting that patients receiving the higher dose had a greater likelihood of having a dry macula at any given exam. This concept was further explored in the VIEW trials where aflibercept 2 mg every 8 weeks produced comparable gains to 0.5 mg every 4 weeks. Furthermore, the two 2 mg aflibercept arms required 4.1 and 4.2 injections during the second year of the VIEW compared to 4.6 injections by the 0.5 mg aflibercept arm [12]. So during the 3 month capped PRN phase of the study, patients receiving the higher dose of aflibercept appeared to experience a longer duration of clinical action than those receiving the lower dose.

Many physicians inject more than the standard 0.05 ml dose of the anti-VEGF drugs with the hope that more molecules will lead to a better therapeutic response. Current data suggests that this strategy does little to improve the maximum number of letters gained, but rather it slightly prolongs the duration of drug action. For example, increasing the volume from 0.05 ml to 0.07 ml probably prolongs the duration of action by 2 to 4 days whereas doubling the volume to 0.1 ml extends the duration by only 5 to 8 days.

The pivotal phase 3 exudative AMD trials showed that most patients respond well to monthly anti-VEGF therapy. Bevacizumab, ranibizumab, and aflibercept each prevent moderate vision loss (> 15 letters of vision) in approximately 95% of patients [5,9,10,77]. Furthermore, between 30% and 40% of patients achieve an improvement of at least 15 letters and the majority of patients demonstrate some improvement in vision. This is generally accompanied by a decrease in the thickness of the retina by -130 μm to -230 μm [5]. Though improvement in vision and decrease in macular thickness are not co-dependent functions, there exists a high correlation between the two.

Most physicians view drying of the macula as the most important treatment endpoint. They make retreatment decisions based primarily upon macular thickness and the presence of intraretinal, subretinal and sub-RPE fluid. Despite the prevailing belief that most patients achieve dry maculas throughout the course of their treatment, trials suggest that only a minority of patients actually maintain a dry macula through 1 year [61]. The CATT (Comparison of Age-Related Macular Degeneration Treatment Trials) showed that 45% of patients receiving monthly ranibizumab remained dry but fewer than 26% of patients receiving monthly bevacizumab or PRN injections of either drug remained dry.

A couple of conclusions can be reached from these observations. First, when used in similar treatment regimens, ranibizumab "dries" the macula better than bevacizumab. Though the exact reason for this is not completely understood, ranibizumab's superior binding affinity for VEGF and its ability to prevent VEGF-mediated activation of vascular endothelial cells probably maintains a dry macula. Secondly, additional drug (beyond the standard doses of 0.05 ml) does little to increase the number of letters of vision gained. Rather, it prolongs the drug's duration of action, although by only a few days.

Standard Strategies

In most of the pivotal AMD trials, patients were treated with monthly anti-VEGF injections. [3,4,10,11] This was based on experimental data which suggested that intravitreal injections of ranibizumab would maintain sufficiently high intraocular concentrations to inhibit VEGF activity for 1 month. The MARINA [77] and ANCHOR [9] trials, therefore, compared monthly injections to observation and photodynamic therapy respectively. Subsequent trials (CATT [61], IVAN [13] and HARBOR [10]) treated patients with monthly injections of ranibizumab and bevacizumab while also randomizing patients to treatment arms with monthly examinations and as-needed injections. These trials determined that monthly injections of bevacizumab or ranibizumab improved vision by an average of +5.0 to +10.2 letters at one year (Table 1).

The VIEW trials [5] reiterated a couple of important treatment concepts regarding anti-VEGF treatment of AMD. First, the monthly use of a much higher affinity anti-VEGF drug (aflibercept) in a typical study population does not lead to greater gains in vision. This suggests that maximum visual improvement with anti-VEGF monotherapy has hit a therapeutic "ceiling". Future high-affinity anti-VEGF drugs may be useful for treating a small subset of poor responders but they will not be able to produce superior across-the-board improvements in visual acuity.

Second, the use of a high affinity agent may produce a prolonged treatment effect (as seen in the aflibercept 2 mg q8week arms) as predicted by mathematical modeling [83]. Future anti-VEGF drugs will need to differentiate themselves by prolonging the duration of action rather than by increasing the magnitude of their peak effect.

Though pivotal anti-VEGF drug trials featured protocols with monthly injections, most physicians attempt to individualize treatment according to the needs of each patient. This idea originated when physicians realized that some patients responded well to fewer than monthly intraocular injections. They knew that if proven effective, individualized treatment would lead to fewer injections, lower costs, greater physician availability and fewer patient visits.

The first trial to evaluate individualized therapy was the PrONTO study [57]. Patients were examined monthly and treated with ranibizumab when they had persistent or new fluid, new hemorrhage, an increase in macular thickness or a decrease in visual acuity. At two years, patients received an average of 9.9 injections while gaining an average of +11.1 letters and experiencing -212 μm of macular thinning.

Table 1. Results from the major exudative age-related macular degeneration trials are listed

TRIALS	DRUG(S)	RESULTS
Age-related macular degeneration		
ANCHOR MARINA PrONTO PIER HARBOR	Ranibizumab	• Monthly ranibizumab, bevacizumab and aflibercept produce similar visual gains (7 to 11 letters). • 95% of eyes lose fewer than 15 letters and 80% show improved vision. • Quarterly dosing leads to poor gains in vision.
CATT	Ranibizumab and Bevacizumab	• Bevacizumab and ranibizumab produce similar visual results. • Monthly exams with as-needed injections produce visual gains similar to monthly injections.
VIEW	Aflibercept and Ranibizumab	• Aflibercept q2months is similar to monthly ranibizumab. • Non-responders may be treated by changing drugs, increasing injection frequency or combining with photodynamic therapy.

These impressive results exceeded those of any of the monthly treatment trials and were attributed to the fact that patients were highly compliant and monitored closely throughout the study. Subsequent trials with PRN arms produced impressive gains in vision but all consistently fell short (though generally not statistically significant) of those achieved with monthly injections [10,13,61].

Induction regimens varied from single injections [61] to 3 injections [13] with each retreatment. The need for a 3 injection induction and/or re-induction series is unclear. The differences in vision between the monthly and PRN arms in the IVAN trial [13], which mandated 3 monthly injections for each treatment, were less than those seen in the CATT, where only single injections were given. However, patients in the second year of the CATT who were switched from monthly to PRN injections lost an average of -2.4 letters [61].

This suggested that even a "1-year loading regimen" did not alter the long-term course of the disease. Furthermore, PRN treated patients in IVAN and CATT required similar numbers of injections during the first year [13,61].

Most physicians actually use a treat-and-extend protocol for the majority of patients. According to this strategy, patients are initially treated monthly then, if the macula is dry, the treatment interval is extended by 2 weeks each subsequent visit. This continues until subretinal fluid or macular thickening recurs, at which time the treatment interval is shortened to what had been already determined to be an effective interval. Results with this strategy have varied according to the CNVM subtype [22,23,38]. Nonetheless, it remains an attractive strategy because, unlike the PRN strategy, it should require fewer visits to the physician's office. The ongoing LUCAS Trial (Norway) has enrolled patients in parallel treat-and-extend arms with ranibizumab and bevacizumab.

Physicians are often challenged with eyes that respond incompletely to monthly anti-VEGF therapy. These eyes have worsening subretinal and macular fluid during the course of treatment or persistent fluid despite monthly injections. As mentioned earlier in this chapter, increasing the dose of an anti-VEGF drug does little to improve efficacy in these difficult-to-treat eyes. The most common approach to these eyes is to switch anti-VEGF drugs. Published reports show that switching from bevacizumab to ranibizumab (Figure 2) or from ranibizumab to bevacizumab may help these non-responders. Though these studies are uncontrolled, more studies suggest that switching from ranibizumab to bevacizumab is beneficial [2,20,49,50,55,80]. This may reflect the fact that bevacizumab is the drug of choice for most physicians so more patients are initially treated with bevacizumab. However, it may also reflect the fact that ranibizumab has a higher binding affinity for VEGF which may provide a superior effect in the most difficult to treat eyes.

Since aflibercept has a much higher binding affinity for VEGF than has either bevacizumab or ranibizumab, many physicians thought that this would lead to greater improvements in visual acuity. The VIEW trials, however, showed that vision gains in the various aflibercept arms were comparable to those in the ranibizumab arms [5]. Furthermore, these gains were comparable to those attained in other pivotal AMD studies with anti-VEGF drugs (i.e. MARINA, ANCHOR, HARBOR, CATT) [9,10,61,77]. These data, accumulated from drugs with substantially different VEGF affinities, suggest that the VEGF-binding affinity of a drug has little effect on the visual improvement experienced by the average patient in a controlled trial.

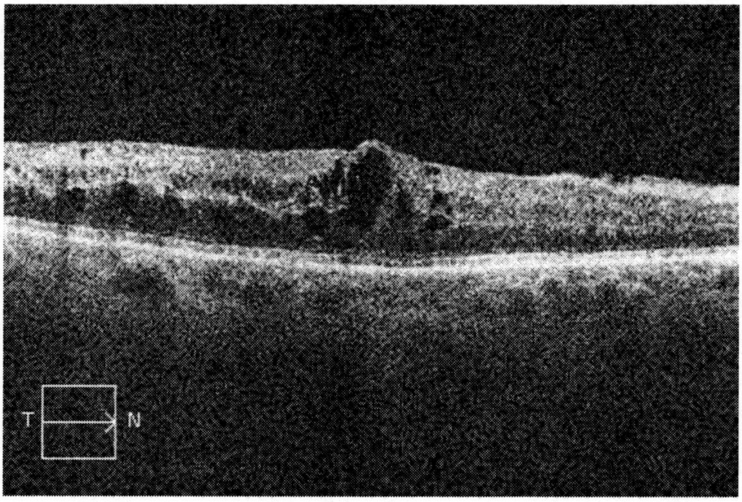

Figure 2.a. The SD-OCT scan shows persistent macular edema in a patient receiving monthly bevacizumab.

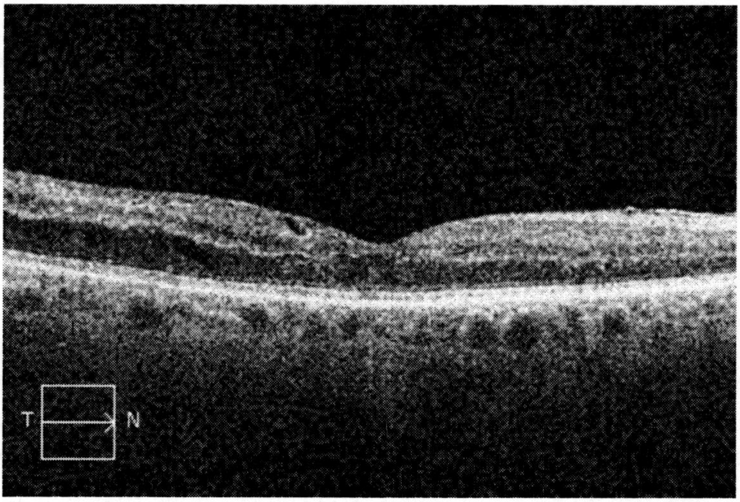

Figure 2.b. The scan shows significant resolution of edema 4 weeks after a first injection of ranibizumab.

Despite the excellent results in pivotal trials, we still see a small number of patients that respond poorly to initial anti-VEGF therapy but respond favorably after changing to a higher affinity drug. Since FDA approval, aflibercept has not been available long enough to determine if its duration of action matches the results from the VIEW trials. However, aflibercept appears very effective as a salvage drug for patients who respond poorly to monthly injections of bevacizumab and ranibizumab. The most reasonable explanation for this phenomenon involves its very high affinity for VEGF. Aflibercept may better neutralize diffusible VEGF, thereby improving leakage and decreasing residual fluid. Alternatively, the fact that, unlike bevacizumab and ranibizumab, aflibercept neutralizes both VEGF-B and placental growth factor may be important in these eyes. Finally, it may be that simply changing drugs to avoid an immunological response to the drug is the most important factor.

Some authors suggest that eyes which respond poorly to monthly anti-VEGF injections have inflammatory cytokines and growth factors other than VEGF dominating the neovascular drive [82]. Though this hypothesis is appealing and may explain the poor clinical responses, there is no direct evidence to support it. Since we know that VEGF is both sufficient and necessary for neovascularization, alternative explanations concerning VEGF suppression should be considered. Suppression requires adequate inactivation of soluble VEGF in the proximity of the vascular endothelial cell receptors. This requires that the inhibitory drug diffuse into the peri-vascular space at a sufficiently high concentration. Poor responses may be due to poor penetration of the drug into the perivascular space with unfavorable drug: VEGF concentrations or an abnormally rapid clearance from the eye. If this is correct then higher concentrations or more efficient VEGF binding (represented by a higher binding affinity) should improve the clinical response. Clinically, one would not see a greater peak response (not more macular thinning) but rather a prolonged clinical effect.

Many eyes that show poor clinical responses one month after the intravitreal injections of anti-VEGF drugs actually have good, although brief, clinical responses at one to two weeks. Therefore, these eyes are better characterized as "brief responders" rather than "non-responders". Performing intravitreal injections every 2 weeks, either with sequential bevacizumab injections or with alternating bevacizumab and ranibizumab, can lead to a sustainable clinical response (Figure 3) [84].

This strategy is more effective than monthly injections of either drug even with higher administered doses because it produces higher trough VEGF-binding capacities. Reactivation of the neovascular drive, which coincides with a sub-therapeutic VEGF-binding capacity prior to the subsequent monthly injection, is prevented because of the higher trough levels. Physicians faced with brief responders should consider biweekly anti-VEGF injections rather than increasing the administered dose.

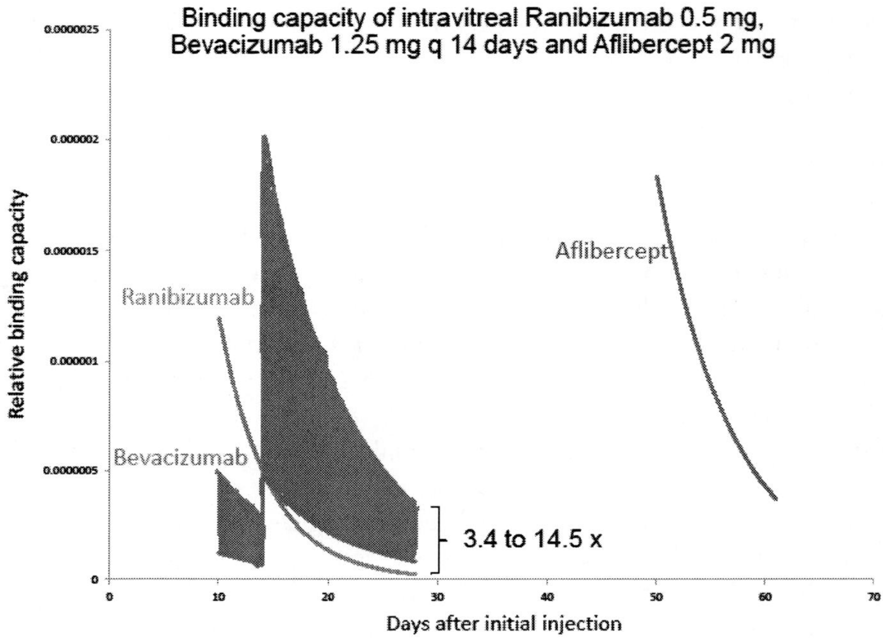

Figure 3. This graph shows the relative VEGF binding capacities of single ranibizumab (0.5 mg) and aflibercept (2 mg), as well as bevacizumab (1.25 mg) given every 14 days. Note that the 1 month binding capacity of high frequency bevacizumab exceeds that of monthly ranibizumab, but both fall short of that produced by aflibercept.

Conclusion

The success of the antibody-based anti-VEGF drugs has established intravitreal anti-VEGF monotherapy as the standard of care for exudative AMD. Nonetheless, new anti-VEGF drugs continue to be developed. Perhaps the most promising is the DARPin MP0112 molecule which has completed phase 2 trials for AMD and diabetic macular edema. Since this drug possesses a high affinity for $VEGF_{165}$ and a surprisingly long intraocular half-life (13.5 days) it promises to deliver a prolonged anti-VEGF effect.

Some physicians advocate combination therapy with corticosteroids and/or photodynamic therapy (PDT) with the belief that this strategy leads to superior gains in vision and fewer treatments. PDT trials have, however, been disappointing as they have not demonstrated superior results over anti-VEGF monotherapy. This has led CMS to consider withdrawing PDT as a “covered therapy” for AMD.

Effective combination therapy will likely await the approval of new drugs which target other (non-VEGF) cellular receptors and pathways. A recent report showed the benefit of adding a platelet derived growth factor inhibitor (fovista, Ophthotech, New York, NY) to monthly ranibizumab therapy. Compared to ranibizumab monotherapy, patients receiving combination therapy experienced superior improvements in vision (+6.5 letters vs. +10.6 letters) and greater regression of the CNVM at 6 months [74]. Several other molecules are also being evaluated.

References

[1] Aiello, L.P., Avery, R.L., Arrigg, P.G., Keyt, B.A., Jampel, H.D., Shah, S.T., Pasquale, L.R., Theime, H., Iwamoto, M.A., Park, J.E., Nguyen, H.V., Aiello, L.M., Ferrara, N., King, G.L., (1994). Vascular endothelial growth factor in ocular fluid of patients with diabetic retinopathy and other retinal disorders. *N. Engl. J. Med.* 131(22), 1480-147.

[2] Almony, A., Mansouri, A., Shah, G.K., Blinder, K.J., (2011). Efficacy of intravitreal bevacizumab after unresponsive treatment with intravitreal ranibizumab. *Can. J. Ophthalmol.* 46(2), 182-185.

[3] Avery, R.L., Pearlman, J., Pieramici, D.J., Rabena, M.D., Castellarin, A.A., Nasir, M.A., Giust, M.J., Wendel, R., Patel, A., (2006). Intravitreal bevacizumab (Avastin) in the treatment of proliferative diabetic retinopathy. *Ophthalmology* 113(10), 1695.e1-15.

[4] Bakri, S.J., Snyder, M.R., Reid, J.M., Pulido, J.S., Singh, R.J., (2007). Pharmacokinetics of intravitreal bevacizumab (Avastin). *Ophthalmology* 114, 855-859.

[5] Bayer and Regeneron Report Positive Top-Line Results of Two Phase 3 Studies with VEGF Trap-Eye in Wet Age-related Macular Degeneration. http://investor.regeneron.com/releasedetail.cfm?ReleaseID=552099 Accessed April 13, 2012.

[6] Bridges, E.M., Harris, A.L., (2011). The angiogenic process as a therapeutic target in cancer. *Biochem. Pharmacol.* 81, 1183-1191.

[7] Brown, D.M., Campochiaro, P.A., Singh, R.P., Li, Z., Gray, S., Saroj, N., Rundle, A.C., Rubio, R.G., Murahashi, W.Y., and CRUISE Investigators, (2010). Ranibizumab for macular edema following central retinal vein occlusion. Six month primary end point results of a phase III study. *Ophthalmology* 117, 1124-1133.

[8] Brown, D.M., Heier, J.S., Ciulla, T., Benz, M., Abraham, P., Yancopoulos, G., Stahl, N., Ingerman, A., Vitti, R., Berliner, A.J., Yang, K., Nguyen, Q.D.; CLEAR-IT 2 Investigators, (2011). Primary endpoint results of a phase II study of vascular endothelial growth factor trap-eye in wet age-related macular degeneration. *Ophthalmology* 118, 1089-1097.

[9] Brown, D.M., Kaiser, P.K., Michels, M, Soubrane, G., Heier, J.S., Kim, R.Y, Sy, J.P., Schneider, S.; ANCHOR Study Group, (2006). Ranibizumab versus verteporfin for neovascular age-related macular degeneration. *N. Engl. J. Med.* 355, 1432-1444.

[10] Busbee, B.G., Yee, W., Li, Z., Rubio, R.G. Efficacy and safety of 2.0-mg or 0.5 mg ranibizumab in patients with subfoveal neovascular AMD: HARBOR Study. American Academy of Ophthalmology Annual Meeting, Orlando FL, October 24, 2011.

[11] Byrne, A.M., Bouchier-Hayes, D.J., Harmey, J.H., (2005). Angiogenic and cell survival functions of vascular endothelial growth factor (VEGF). *J. Cell. Mol. Med.* 9, 777-794.

[12] Campochiaro, P.A., Heier, J.S., Feiner, L., and BRAVO investigators, (2010). Ranibizumab for macular edema following branch retinal vein occlusion. Six month primary end point results of a phase III study. *Ophthalmology* 117, 1102-1112.

[13] Chakravarthy, U., Harding, S.P., Rogers, C.A., Downes, S.M., Lotery, A.J., IVAN Study Investigators, (2012). Ranibizumab versus bevacizumab to treat neovascular age-related macular degeneration. One-year findings from the IVAN randomized trial. *Ophthalmology* 119, 1399-1411.

[14] Christofordis, J.B., Carlton, M.M., Knopp, M.V., Hinkle, G.H., (2011). Pet/CT imaging of I-124-radiolabeled bevacizumab and ranibizumab after intravitreal injection in a rabbit model. *Invest. Ophthalmol. Vis. Sci.* 52, 5899-5903.

[15] Connolly, D.T., Heuvelman, D.M., Nelson, R., Olander, J.V., Eppley, B.L., Delfino, J.J., Siegel, N.R., Leimgruber, R.M., Feder, J., (1989). Tumor vascular permeability factor stimulates endothelial cell growth and angiogenesis. *J. Clin. Invest.* 84, 1470-1478.

[16] de Vries, C., Escobedo, J.A., Ueno, H., Houck, K., Ferrara, N., Williams, L.T., (1992). The fms-like tyrosine kinase, a receptor for vascular endothelial growth factor. *Science* 255, L989-991.

[17] Diago, T., Pulido, J.S., Molina, J.R., Collett, L.C., Link, T.P., Ryan, E.H. Jr., (2008). Ranibizumab combined with low-dose sorafenib for

exudative age-related macular degeneration. *Mayo Clin. Proc.* 83(2), 231-234.

[18] Dib, E., Maia, M., Longo-Maugeri, I.M., Martins, M.C., Mussalem, J.S., Squaiella, C.C., Penha, F.M., Magalhaes, O. Jr., Rodrigues, E.B., Farah, M.E., (2008). Subretinal bevacizumab detection after intravitreous injection in rabbits. *Invest. Ophthalmol. Vis. Sci.* 49, 1097-1100.

[19] Ding, Y., Huang, Y., Song, N., Gao, X., Yuan, S., Wang, X., Cai, H., Fu, Y., Luo, Y., (2010). NFAT1 mediates placental growth factor-induced myelomonocytic cell recruitment via the induction of TNF-α. *J. Immunol.* 184, 2593-2601.

[20] Ehlers, J.P., Spim, M.J., Shah, C.P., Fenton, G.L., Baker, P.S., Regillo, C.D., Ho, A.C., (2010). Ranibizumab for exudative age-related macular degeneration in eyes previously treated with alternative vascular endothelial growth factor inhibitors. *Ophthalmic Surg. Lasers Imaging* 4(12), 182-189.

[21] Elicieri, B.P., Paul, R., Schwartzberg, P.L., Hood, J.D., Leng, J., Cheresh, D.A., (1999). Selective requirement for Src kinases during VEGF-induced angiogenesis and vascular permeability. *Mol. Cell.* 4, 915-924.

[22] Engelbert, M., Zweifel, S.A., Freund, K.B., (2009). Treat and extend dosing of intravitreal antivascular growth factor therapy for type 3 neovascularization/retinal angiomatous proliferation. *Retina* 29(10), 1424-1431.

[23] Engelbert, M., Zweifel, S.A., Freund, K.B., (2010). Long-term follow-up for type 1 (subretinal pigment epithelium) neovascularization using a modified "treat and extend" dosing regimen of intravitreal antivascular endothelial growth factor therapy. *Retina* 30(9), 1368-1375.

[24] Ferrara, N., Damico, L., Shams, N., Lowman, H., Kim, R., (2006) Development of ranibizumab, an anti-vascular endothelial growth factor antigen binding fragment, as therapy for neovascular age-related macular degeneration. *Retina* 26, 859-870.

[25] Ferrara, N., Davis-Smyth, T., (1987). The biology of vascular endothelial growth factor. *Endocr. Rev.* 18, 4-25.

[26] Ferrara, N.P., Gerber, H-P., LeCouter, J., (2003). The biology of VEGF and its receptors. *Nat. Med.* 9(6), 669-676.

[27] Ferrara, N., Henzel, W.J., (1989). Pituitary follicular cells secrete a novel heparin-binding growth factor specific for vascular endothelial cells. *Biochem. Biophys. Res. Commun.* 161, 851-858.

[28] Folkman, J., (1971). Tumor angiogenesis: therapeutic implications. *N. Engl. J. Med.* 285, 1182-1186.
[29] Folkman, J., Shing, Y., (1992). Angiogenesis. *J. Biol. Chem.* 267, 10931-10934.
[30] Fujisawa, H., Kitsukawa, T., Kawakami, A., Takagi, S., Shimizu, M., Hirata, T., (1997). Roles of a neuronal cell-surface molecule, neuropilin, in nerve fiber fasciculation and guidance. *Cell. Tissue Res.* 290, 465-470.
[31] Furfine, E., Coppi, A., Koehler-Stec, E., Zimmer, E., Tu, W., Struble, C., (2006). Pharmacokinetics and ocular tissue penetration of VEGF Trap after intravitreal injections in rabbits. *Invest. Ophthalmol. Vis. Sci.* 47, E-abstract 1430.
[32] Gaudreault, J., Damico, L.A., Haughney, P.C., (2004). A pharmacokinetic model describing ocular and systemic disposition of ranibizumab in rabbits. *Invest. Ophthalmol. Vis. Sci.* 45, ARVO E-Abstract 1854.
[33] Gaudreault, J., Fei, D., Rusit, J., Suboc, P., Shiu, V., (2005). Preclinical pharmacokinetics of ranitbizumab (rhuFabV2) after a single intravitreal administration. *Invest. Ophthalmol. Vis. Sci.* 46, 726-733.
[34] Gaudreault, J., Webb, W., Van Hoy, M., (1999). Pharmacokinetics and retinal distribution of AMD rhufab V2 after intravitreal administration in rabbits. *AAPS Pharm. Sci.* (supp 1), 3207.
[35] Good, T.J., Kimura, A.E., Mandava, Kahook, M.Y., (2011). Sustained elevation of intraocular pressure after intravitreal injections of anti-VEGF agents. *Br. J. Ophthalmol.* 95, 1111-1114.
[36] Gordon, M.S., Margolin, K., Talpaz, M., Sledge, G.W. Jr., Holmgren, E., Benjamin, R., Stalter, S., Shak, S., Adelman, D., (2001). Phase 1 safety and pharmacokinetic study of recombinant human anti-vascular endothelial growth factor in patients with advanced cancer. *J. Clin. Oncol.* 19, 843-850.
[37] Guo, D., Jia, Q., Song, H.Y., Warren, R.S., Donner, D.B., (1995). Vascular endothelial cell growth factor promotes tyrosine phosphorylation of mediators of signal transduction that contain SH2 domains. Association with endothelial cell proliferation. *J. Biol. Chem.* 270, 6729-6733.
[38] Gupta, O.P., Shienbaum, G., Patel, A.H., Fecarotta, C., Kaiser, R.S., Regillo, C.D., (2010). A treat and extend regimen using ranibizumab for neovascular age-related macular degeneration clinical and economic impact. *Ophthalmology* 117(11), 2134-2140.

[39] Haughney, J., Lowe, A., Kearns, J. Clinical pharmacokinetics of ranibizumab (Lucentis) in subjects with AMD. ARVO abstract, May 2, 2005.

[40] Heiduschka, P., Fietz, H., Hofmeister, S., Schultheiss, S., Mack, A.F., Peters, S., Ziemssen, F., Niggemann, B., Julien, S., Bartz-Schmidt, K.U., Schraermeyer, U., Tübingen Bevacizumab Study Group, (2007). Penetration of bevacizumab through the retina after intravitreal injection in the monkey. *Invest. Ophthalmol. Vis. Sci.* 48, 2814-2823.

[41] Heier, J.S., Antoszyk, A.N., Pavan, P.R., Leff, S.R., Rosenfeld, P.J., Ciulla, T.A., Dreyer, R.F., Gentile, R.C., Sy, J.P., Hantsbarger, G., Shams, N., (2006). Ranibizumab for treatment of neovascular age-related macular degeneration: a phase I/II multicenter, controlled, multidose study. *Ophthalmology* 113(4), 633.e1-4.

[42] Heier, J.S., Boyer, D., Nguyen, Q.D., Marcus, D., Roth, D.B., Yancopoulos, G., Stahl, N., Ingerman, A., Vitti, R., Berliner, A.J., Yang, K., Brown, D.M., CLEAR-IT 2 Investigators, (2011). The 1-year results of CLEAR-IT 2, a phase 2 study of vascular endothelial growth factor trap-eye dosed as-needed after 12-week fixed dosing. *Ophthalmology* 118, 1098-1106.

[43] Holash, J., Davis, S., Papadopoulos, N., et al., (2002). VEGF-Trap: a VEGF blocker with potent antitumor effects. *PNAS* 99(17), 11393-11398.

[44] Houck, K.A., Ferrara, N., Winer, J., Cachianes, G., Li, B., Leung, D.W., (1991). The vascular endothelial growth factor family: identification of a fourth molecular species and characterization of alternative splicing of RNA. *Mol. Endocrinol.* 5, 1806-1814.

[45] Houck, K.A., Leung, D.W., Rowland, A.M., Winer, J., Ferrara, N., (1992). Dual regulation of vascular endothelial growth factor bioavailability by genetic and proteolytic mechanisms. *J. Biol. Chem.* 267, 26031-26037.

[46] Hurwitz, H., Fehrenbacher, L., Novotny, W., Cartwright, T., Hainsworth, J., Heim, W., Berlin, J., Baron, A., Griffing, S., Holmgren, E., Ferrara, N., Fyfe, G., Rogers, B., Kabbinavar, F., (2004). Bevacizumab plus irinotecan, fluorouracil, and leucovorin for metastatic colorectal cancer. *N. Engl. J. Med.* 350(23), 2335-2342.

[47] Ishida, S., Usui, T., Yamashiro, K., Kaji, Y., Amano, S., Ogura, Y., Hida, T., Oguchi, Y., Ambati, J, Miller, J.W., Gragoudas, E.S., Ng, Y.S., D'Amore, P.A., Shima, D.T., Adamis, A.P., (2003). $VEGF_{164}$-mediated

inflammation is required for pathological, but not physiological, ischemia-induced retinal neovascularization. *J. Exp. Med.* 198, 483-489.

[48] Kaiser, P.K., (2006). Antivascular endothelial growth factor agents and their development: therapeutic implications in ocular diseases. *Am. J. Ophthalmol.* 142, 660-668.

[49] Kaiser, R.S., Gupta, O.P., Regillo, C.D., Ho, A.C., Fineman, M.S., Vander, J.F., McNamara, J.A., Brown, G.C., (2012). Ranibizumab for eyes previously treated with pegaptanib or bevacizumab without clinical response. *Ophthalmic Surg. Lasers Imaging* 43(1), 13-19.

[50] Karagiannis, D.A., Ladas, I.D., Parikakis, E., Georgalas, I., Kotsolis, A., Amariotakis, G., Soumplis, V., Mitropoulos, P., (2009). Changing from bevacizumab to ranibizumab in age-related macular degeneration. Is it safe? Clin. Interv. Aging 4, 457-461.

[51] Karkkainan, M.J., Makinen, T., Alitalo, K., (2002). Lymphatic endothelium: a new frontier of metastasis research. *Nat. Cell. Biol.* 4, E2-E5.

[52] Klettner, A., Roider, J., (2009). Treating age-related macular degeneration – interaction of VEGF-antagonists with their target. *Mini. Rev. Med. Chem.* 9, 1127-1135.

[53] Krohne, T.U., Eter, N., Holz, F.G., Meyer, C.H., (2008). Intraocular pharmacokinetics of bevacizumab after a single intravitreal injection in humans. *Am. J. Ophthalmol.* 146(4), 508-512.

[54] Kuroki, M., Voest, E.E., Amano, S., Beerepoot, L.V., Takashima, S., Tolentino, M., Kim, R.Y., Rohan, R.M., Colby, K.A., Yeo, K.T., Adamis, A.P., (1996). Reactive oxygen intermediates increase vascular endothelial growth factor expression in vitro and in vivo. *J. Clin. Invest.* 98, 495-504.

[55] Labriola, L.T., Sadda, S.R., (2011). Rapid resolution of macular edema associated with central retinal vein occlusion using ranibizumab after failure with multiple bevacizumab injections. *Semin. Ophthalmol.* 26(6), 387-391.

[56] Lähteenvuo, J.E., Lähteenvuo, M.T., Kivelä, A., Rosenlew, C., Falkevall, A., Klar, J., Keifura, T., Rissanen, T.T., Vähäkangas, E., Korpisalo, P., Enholm, B., Carmeliet, P., Alitalo, K., Eriksson, U., Ylä-Herttuala, S. , (2009). Vascular endothelial growth factor-B induces myocardium-specific angiogenesis and arteriogenesis via vascular endothelial growth factor receptor-1 and neuropilin receptor-1-dependent mechanisms. *Circulation* 119(6), 845-856.

[57] Lalwani, G.A., Rosenfeld, P.J., Fung, A.E., Dubovy, S.R., Michels, S., Feuer, W., Davis, J.L., Flynn, H.W. Jr., Esquiabro, M., (2009). A variable-dosing regimen with intravitreal ranibizumab for neovascular age-related macular degeneration: year 2 of the PrONTO Study. *Am. J. Ophthalmol.* 148, 43-58.

[58] Lopez, P.F., Sippy, B.D., Lambert, H.M., Thach, A.B., Hinton, D.R., (1996). Tran differentiated retinal pigment epithelial cells are immunoreactive for vascular endothelial growth factor in surgically excised age-related macular degeneration-related choroidal neovascular membranes. *Invest. Ophthalmol. Vis. Sci.* 37, 855-868.

[59] Lu, M., Adamis, A.P., (2006). Molecular biology of choroidal neovascularization. *Ophthalmol. Clin. N. Am.* 19, 323-334.

[60] Lu, M., Kuroki, M., Amano, S., Tolentino, M., Keough, K., Kim, I., Bucala, R., Adamis, A.P., (1998). Advanced glycation end products increase retinal vascular endothelial growth factor expression. *J. Clin. Invest.* 101, 1219-1224.

[61] Martin, D.F., Maguire, M.G., Ying, G-S, (2011). Ranibizumab and bevacizumab for neovascular age-related macular degeneration. *N. Engl. J. Med.* 364, 1897-1908.

[62] McColm, J.R., Geisen, P., Hartnett, M.E., (2004). VEGF isoforms and their expression after a single episode of hypoxia or repeated fluctuations between hyperoxia and hypoxia: relevance to clinical ROP. *Mol. Vis.* 10, 512-550.

[63] Meyer, C.H., Krohne, T.U., Holz, F.G., (2011). Intraocular pharmacokinetics after a single intravitreal injection of 1.5 mg versus 3.0 mg of bevacizumab in humans. *Retina* 31(9), 1877-1884.

[64] Michaelson, I.C., (1948). The mode of development of the vascular system of the retina with some observations on its significance for certain retinal disorders. *Trans. Ophthalmol. Soc. UK* 68, 1625-1710.

[65] Mordenti, J., Cuthbertson, R.A., Ferrara, N., Thomsen, K., Berleau, L., Licko, V., Allen, P.C., Valverde, C.R., Meng, Y.G., Fei, D.T., Fourre, K.M., Ryan, A.M., (1999). Comparisons of the intraocular tissue distribution, pharmacokinetics, and safety of ^{125}I-labeled full-length and Fab antibodies in rhesus monkeys following intravitreal administration. *Toxicol. Pathol.* 27, 536-544.

[66] Neufeld, G., Cohen, T., Gengrinovitch, S., Poltorak, Z, (1999). Vascular endothelial growth factor (VEGF) and its receptors. *FASEB J.* 13, 9-22.

[67] Ng, E.W.M., Shima, D.T., Calias, P., Cunningham, E.T. Jr., Guyer, D.R., Adamis, A.P., (2006). Pegaptanib, a targeted anti-VEGF aptamer for ocular vascular disease. *Nat. Rev. Drug Disc*. 5, 123-132.

[68] Nguyen, Q.D., Shah, S.M., Browning, D.J., Hudson, H., Sonkin, P., Hariprasad, S.M., Kaiser, P., Slakter, J.S., Haller, J., Do, D.V., Mieler, W.F., Chu, K., Yang, K., Ingerman, A., Vitti, R.L., Berliner, A.J., Cedarbaum, J.M., Campochiaro, P.A., (2009). A phase I study of intravitreal vascular endothelial growth factor trap-eye in patients with neovascular age-related macular degeneration. *Ophthalmology* 116, 2141-2148.

[69] Nguyen, Q.D., Shah, S.M., Hafiz, G., Quinlan, E., Sung, J., Chu, K., Cedarbaum, J.M., Campochiaro, P.A., CLEAR-AMD 1 Study Group, (2006). A phase I trial of an IV-administered vascular endothelial growth factor trap for treatment in patients with choroidal neovascularization due to age-related macular degeneration. *Ophthalmology* 113, 1522-1532.

[70] Nomoto, H., Shiraga, F., Kuno, N., Kimura, E., Fujii, S., Shinomiya, K., Nugent, A.K., Hirooka, K., Baba, T., (2009). Pharmacokinetics of bevacizumab after topical, subconjunctival, and intravitreal administration in rabbits. *Invest. Ophthalmol. Vis. Sci.* 50, 4807-4813.

[71] Olofsson, B., Korpelainen, E., Pepper, M.S., Mandriota, S.J., Aase, K., Kumar, V., Gunji, Y., Jeltsch, M.M., Shibuya, M., Alitalo, K., Eriksson, U., (1998). Vascular endothelial growth factor B (VEGFB) binds to VEGF receptor-1 and regulates plasminogen activator activity in endothelial cells. *Proc. Natl. Acad. Sci.* 95, 11709-11714.

[72] Papadopoulos, N., Martin, J., Ruan, Q., Rafique, A., Rosconi, M.P., Shi, E., Pyles, E.A., Yancopoulos, G.D., Stahl, N., Wiegand, S.J., (2012). Binding and neutralization of vascular endothelial growth factor (VEGF) and related ligands by VEGF Trap, ranibizumab and bevacizumab. *Angiogenesis* Feb 3, [Epub ahead of print].

[73] Park, J.E., Keller, G-A., Ferrara, N., (1993). The vascular endothelial growth factor (VEGF) isoforms: differential disposition into the subepithelial extracellular matrix and bioactivity of ECM-bound VEGF. *Mol. Biol. Cell*. 4, 131-1326.

[74] Press release: anti-PEDF agent combined with Lucentis beats anti-VEGF monotherapy for exudative AMD. http://www.news-medical.net/news /20120614/Ophthoteche28099s-Fovista-anti-PDGF-combination-therapy-superior-to-Lucentis-for-wet-AMD.aspx. Accessed 9-11-2012.

[75] Presta, L.G., Chen, H., O'Connor, S.J., Chisholm, V., Meng, Y.G., Krummen, L., Winkler, M., Ferrara, N.., (1997). Humanization of an anti-vascular endothelial growth factor monoclonal antibody for the therapy of solid tumors and other disorders. *Cancer Res.* 57, 4593-4599.

[76] Rakic, J.M., Lambert, V., Devy, L., Lutten, A., Carmeliet, P., Claes, C., Nguyen, L., Foidart, J.M., Noël, A., Munaut, C., (2003). Placental growth factor, a member of the VEGF family, contributes to the development of choroidal neovascularization. *Invest. Ophthalmol. Vis. Sci.* 44(7), 3186-3193.

[77] Rosenfeld, P.J., Brown, D.M., Heier, J.S., Boyer, D.S., Kaiser, P.K., Chung, C.Y., Kim, R.Y., MARINA Study Group, (2006). Ranibizumab for age-related macular degeneration. *N. Engl. J. Med.* 355, 1419-1431.

[78] Rosenfeld, P.J., Heier, J.S., Hantsbarger, G., Shams, N., (2006). Tolerability and efficacy of multiple escalating doses of ranibizumab (Lucentis) for neovascular age-related macular degeneration. *Ophthalmology* 113(4), 623.e1.

[79] Senger, D.R., Galli, S.J., Dvorak, A.M., Perruzzi, C.A., Harvey, V.S., Dvorak, H.F., (1983). Tumor cells secrete a vascular permeability factor that promotes accumulation of ascites fluid. *Science* 12, 983-985.

[80] Spaide, R.F., Chang, L.K., Klancik, J.M., Yannuzzi, L.A., Sorenson, J., Slakter, J.S., Freund, K.B., Klein, R., (2009). Prospective study of intravitreal ranibizumab as a treatment for decreased visual acuity secondary to central retinal vein occlusion. *Am. J. Ophthalmol.* 147(2), 298-306.

[81] Stewart, M.W., (2011). What are the half-lives of ranibizumab and aflibercept (VEGF Trap-eye) in human eyes? Calculations with a mathematical model. *Eye Reports* 1(1), e5.

[82] Stewart, M.W., (2012). Clinical and differential utility of VEGF inhibitors in wet age-related macular degeneration: focus on aflibercept. *Clin. Ophthalmol.* 6, 1175-1186.

[83] Stewart, M.W., Rosenfeld, P.J., (2008). Predicted biological activity of intravitreal VEGF Trap. *Br. J. Ophthalmol.* 92(5), 667-668.

[84] Stewart, M.W., Rosenfeld, P.J., Penha, F.M., Wang, F., Yehoshua, Z., Bueno-Lopez, E., Lopez, P.F., (2012). Pharmacokinetic rationale for dosing every 2 weeks versus 4 weeks with intravitreal ranibizumab, bevacizumab, and aflibercept (vascular endothelial growth factor trap-eye). *Retina* 32(3), 343-357.

[85] Takahashi, T., Ueno, H., Shibuya, M., (1999). VEGF activates protein kinase C-dependent, but Ras-independent Raf-MEF-MAP kinase

pathway for DNA synthesis in primary endothelial cells. *Oncogene* 18, 2221-2230.

[86] Terman, B.I., Carrion, M.E., Kovacs, E., Rasmussen, B.A., Eddy, R.L., Shows, T.B., (1991). Identification of a new endothelial cell growth factor receptor tyrosine kinase. *Oncogene* 6, 1677-1683.

[87] Tew, W.P., Gordon, M., Murren, J., Dupont, J., Pezzulli, S., Aghajanian, C., Sabbatini, P., Mendelson, D., Schwartz, L., Gettinger, S., Psyrri, A., Cedarbaum, J.M., Spriggs, D.R., (2010). Phase 1 study of aflibercept administered subcutaneously to patients with advanced solid tumors. *Clin. Cancer Res.* 16, 358-366.

[88] The Diabetic Retinopathy Clinical Research Network, (2010). Randomized trial evaluating ranibizumab plus prompt or deferred laser or triamcinolone plus prompt laser for diabetic macular edema. *Ophthalmology* 117, 1064-1077.

[89] Tischer, E., Mitchell, R., Hartman, T., Silva, M., Gospodarowicz, D., Fiddes, J.C., Abraham, J.A., (1991). The human gene for vascular endothelial growth factor. Multiple protein forms are encoded through alternative exon splicing. *J. Biol. Chem.* 266, 11947-11954.

[90] Two Year Results of Phase 3 Studies with EYLEA™ (aflibercept) Injection in wet AMD Show Sustained Improvement in Visual Acuity. http://investor.regeneron.com/releasedeta.

[91] Van Cutsem, E., Tabernero, J., Lakomy, R., (2011). ZALTRAP™ (aflibercept) Significantly Improved Survival in Previously Treated Metastatic Colorectal Cancer Patients. *Ann.Oncol.* 22(suppl 5), v18.

[92] Wang, H,, Keiser, A., (1998). Vascular endothelial growth factor upregulates the expression of matrix metalloproteinases in vascular smooth muscle cells: role of flt-1. *Circ. Res.* 83, 832-840.

[93] Yancopoulos, G.D., Davis, S., Gale, N.W., Rudge, J.S., Wiegand, S.J., Holash, J., (2000). Vascular-specific growth factors and blood vessel formation. *Nature* 407, 242-248.

[94] Yu, L., Liang, X.H., Ferrara, N., (2011). Comparing protein VEGF inhibitors: in vitro biological studies. Biochem. Biophys. Res. Commun. 408, 276-281.

[95] Zhong, X., Huang, H., Shen, J., Zacchingna, S., Zentilin, L., Giacca, M., Vinores, S.A., (2011). Vascular endothelial growth factor-B gene transfer exacerbates retinal and choroidal neovascularization and vasopermeability without promoting inflammation. *Mol. Vis.* 17, 492-507.

[96] Zhu, Q., Zeimssen, F., Henke-Fahle, S., Tatar, O., Szuman, P., Aisenbrey, S., Schneiderhan-Marra, N., Xu, X., Tübingen Bevacizumab Study Group, (2008). Vitreous levels of bevacizumab and vascular endothelial growth factor-A in patients with choroidal neovascularization. *Ophthalmology* 115, 1750-1755.

In: Recent Advances in Ophthalmology Research ISBN: 978-1-62808-021-6
Editor: Galina Dimitrova

Chapter 2

Recent Advances in Ocular Blood Flow Research

Galina Dimitrova[1,*] ***and Satoshi Kato***[2]
[1]Department of Ophthalmology, Medical School
"Goce Delčev" University, Štip, Macedonia
[2]Department of Ophthalmology
University of Tokyo Hospital, Tokyo, Japan

Abstract

Ocular blood flow research is an important segment in the investigation of ophthalmic physiology and pathophysiology. The ocular vascular system is quite complex to satisfy the metabolic needs of the structures of the eye, and on the other hand not to interfere with the passage of light through the optic media.

The methods of ocular blood flow measurement are many and they investigate different aspects of blood flow in specific vascular beds. We discuss the characteristics of the ocular vascular systems and the current and upgraded methods for measurement of ocular blood flow.

Novel techniques of ocular blood flow measurement are also presented. Although some of the imaging techniques are superior to others concerning their accuracy and imaging options, the complexity of the ocular vascular system requires a multitude of technology to obtain

[*] E-mail: galina@sonet.com.mk.

data from its various vascular segments and their specific circulatory patterns.

Keywords: Ocular blood flow, methods, ophthalmic artery, central retinal artery, central retinal vein, ciliary artery

Introduction

The investigation of ocular blood flow has been an important segment of ophthalmic research in patients with ocular and systemic pathology, as well as in healthy subjects. The transparency of the ocular optical system enables the clinician to observe the vascular system of the retina directly. It also enables direct measurement of the retinal blood flow through the optical media using various methods of measurement. The direct visibility of the retinal vascular system has facilitated our understanding of the pathogenesis of retinal vascular diseases as well as other ocular and systemic conditions where the retinal blood vessels are involved. However, unresolved issues remain about the validity of the methods that evaluate various aspects of retinal blood flow. On the other hand, uveal and orbital blood flow is even harder to estimate than retinal blood flow regarding the fact that in normal conditions the uveal and orbital vascular systems cannot be visualized directly.

The ocular vascular system has some specific characteristics that must be considered when evaluating blood flow in its various segments. The methods of blood flow measurement investigate different aspects of blood flow in specific parts of the vascular system (tissue, capillary, venules, and arterioles).

This chapter discusses the characteristics of the ocular vascular system and ocular blood flow. The methods of ocular blood flow measurement will be reviewed with an update of the recent improvements and novel techniques of ocular blood flow measurement.

The Ocular Vascular System

The main blood supply to the eye and orbit is through the ophthalmic artery (a branch of the internal carotid artery). (Figure 1) The venous blood outflow from the eye and orbit is mainly done through the superior and inferior ophthalmic veins. (Figure 2)

After branching from the internal carotid artery within the subarachnoid space, the ophthalmic artery lies within the dural-arachnoid sheath of the optic nerve inside the optic canal. After reaching the orbit, the artery pierces the meningeal sheath and positions a short distance lateral to the optic nerve. The artery lies laterally to the optic nerve for several millimeters and then turns medially towards the medial orbital wall. The ophthalmic artery divides into the supratrochlear and dorsal nasal arteries at the medial end of the upper eyelid.

The following arterial branches emerge from the ophthalmic artery: central retinal artery, lacrimal artery, arterial branches for the bulbomotoric muscles, ciliary arteries (lateral and medial), supraorbital artery, posterior ethmoidal artery, anterior ethmoidal artery, meningeal artery, medial palpebral arteries, supratrochlear, and dorsal nasal artery. (Figure 1)

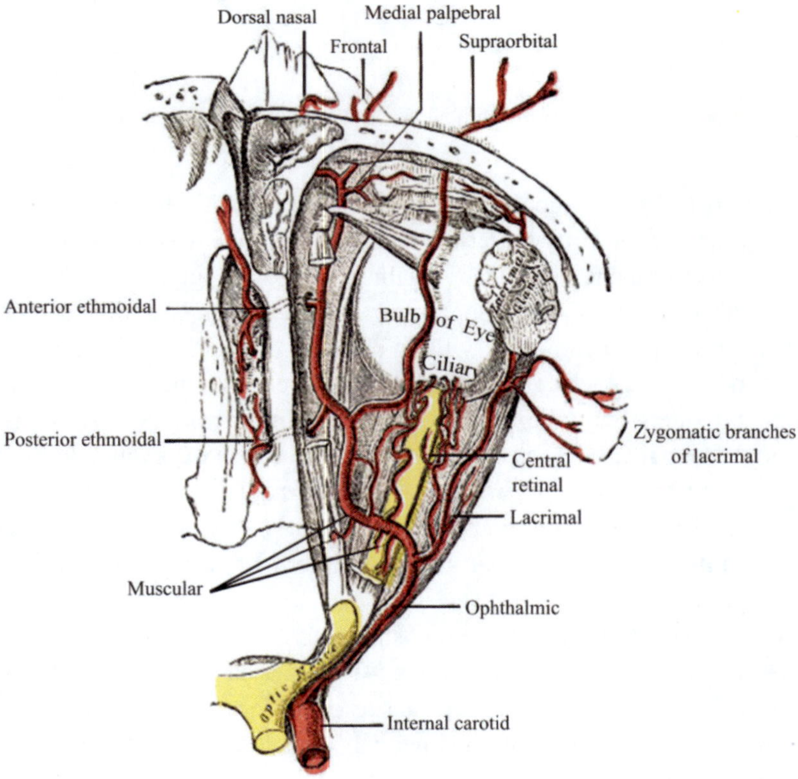

Figure 1. The ophthalmic artery (from Henry Gray. Anatomy of the Human Body, 20th edition).

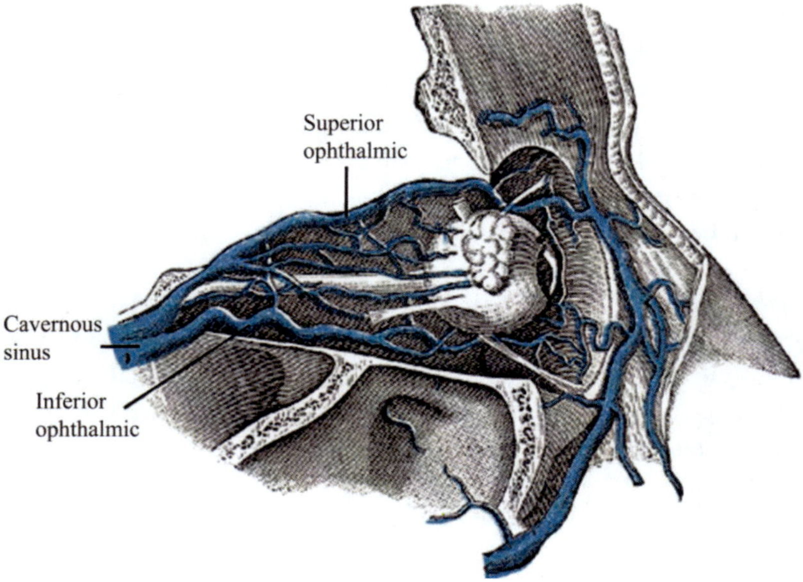

Figure 2. The intraorbital veins (from Henry Gray. Anatomy of the Human Body, 20th edition).

The arterial blood supply to the eyeball is provided by the central retinal artery, the posterior ciliary arteries, and the anterior ciliary artery (branch of the muscular branches of the ophthalmic artery). (Figure 3A) The central retinal artery provides blood supply to the inner segments of the retina. It arises from the ophthalmic artery lying closely to the optic nerve. About 1 cm behind the eyeball, the central retinal artery pierces the optic nerve meningeal sheath and enters the optic nerve where it assumes a central position next to the central retinal vein. The central retinal artery enters the eyeball through the lamina cribrosa where it branches in two main (superior and inferior branches). The two main branches then split to form temporal superior, temporal inferior, nasal superior and nasal inferior branches that supply each quadrant of the retina.

The ciliary arteries provide blood supply to the uvea and to the outer third of the retina. (Figure 3A and Figure 4) The posterior ciliary arteries are (usually) two: medial and lateral posterior ciliary arteries. The long posterior ciliary arteries pierce the eyeball medially and laterally to the optic nerve. They travel beneath the sclera and the choroid and reach the ciliary body. At the iris margin, they split into superior and inferior branches, which encircle the iris and anastomose with the branches of contralateral long posterior ciliary artery. From the long posterior ciliary arteries, also emerge branches, which anastomose with the branches from the anterior ciliary arteries and form the major arterial circle of the iris. The recurrent branches of the posterior ciliary artery, branches from the major arterial circle of the iris, and from the anterior ciliary artery provide arterial blood to the anterior choroid and anastomose with the branches from the short posterior ciliary arteries at the level of the equator. (Figure 4)

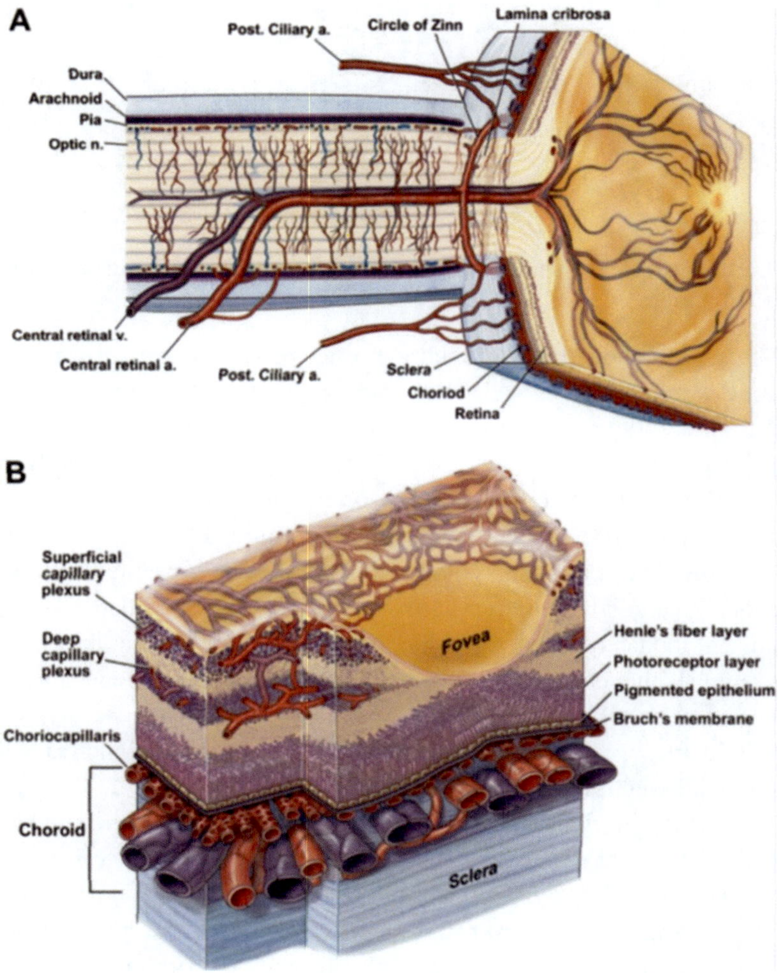

Figure 3.A. A sagital section of the optic nerve and the posterior pole of the eye depicting the central retinal artery and vein, and the short posterior ciliary arteries. B. The vascular system of the retina and choroid (Drawings by Dave Schumick from Anand-Apte and Hollyfield, with permission of Elsevier).

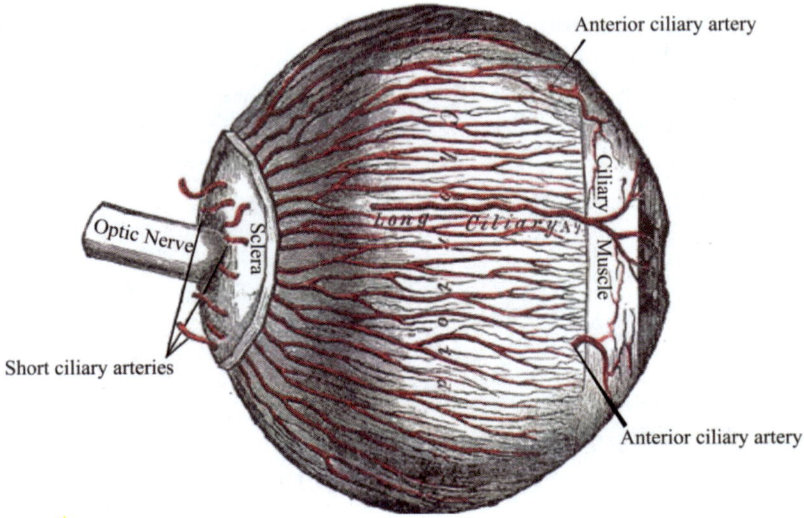

Figure 4. The vascular system of the uvea (from Henry Gray. Anatomy of the Human Body, 20th edition).

The several short posterior ciliary arteries pierce the eyeball very close to the optic nerve. (Figure 3A) They supply the posterior choroid until the equator, where they anastomose with the branches from the posterior ciliary, the major arterial circle of the iris, and the anterior ciliary arteries. Branches from the short posterior ciliary arteries form an anastomotic ring in the sclera around the optic nerve (the circle of Zinn). Arterial branches from the circle of Zinn supply the prelaminar and laminar regions of the optic nerve. Occasionally, a cilioretinal artery arises from the ciliary circulation and enters the retina at the lateral border of the optic nerve. When present, the cilioretinal artery supplies the retinal tissue between the optic disk and the macula.

The anterior ciliary arteries originate from the muscular branches of the ophthalmic artery. (Figure 4) They supply the sclera, the conjunctiva and they also provide branches to the major arterial circle of the iris.

The orbital venous blood drains through the superior and inferior ophthalmic veins to the cavernous sinus. (Figure 2) These veins have no valves. The superior ophthalmic vein is formed by a branch from the supraorbital and a branch from the facial vein. It is larger than the inferior ophthalmic vein and passing posteriorly through the orbital fat it receives venous branches that correspond to the arterial branches of the ophthalmic artery.

The superior ophthalmic vein exits the orbit through the superior orbital fissure. The inferior ophthalmic vein is formed by a venous plexus at the anterior orbital wall. It communicates with branches from the facial vein and branches from the pterygoid plexus. It may either join the superior ophthalmic artery or drain in the sinus cavernosus, or it may pass through the lower part of the inferior orbital fissure and empty into the pterygoid venous plexus.

The central retinal vein is the sole vein that drains the venous blood from the retina. (Figure 3A) It leaves the eyeball through the optic nerve passing at its center. After about 1 cm behind the eyeball, the central retinal vein pierces the meningeal sheaths of the optic nerve and joins the superior ophthalmic vein, or drains directly into the sinus cavernosus.

The choroidal venous blood and most of the venous drainage from the anterior segment are directed posteriorly into the choroid and then into the vortex veins. The two superior vortex veins drain into the superior ophthalmic vein and the two inferior vortex veins drain into the inferior ophthalmic vein.

The Vascular System of the Retina

The retinal vascular system in the human eye had been adapted to satisfy the high metabolic rate of the retinal tissue and to preserve transparency in order not to interfere with the light stimuli. The arterioles that branch from the central retinal artery do not anastomose. Their terminal branches form two layers of capillary networks: superficial and deep capillary plexus. (Figure 3B) The superficial capillary plexus is situated at the ganglion cell layer and the nerve fiber layer. The deep plexus is at the junction between the inner nuclear and the outer plexiform layer. These two networks supply the inner two thirds of the retinal tissue; the outer one third of the retina (photoreceptor layer and retinal pigment epithelium) is supplied with oxygen and nutrients by the choroid.

The capillary networks are absent from the fovea centralis. The foveal avascular zone is approximately 500 μm in diameter. The density of the capillaries is highest at the macula and lowest at the retinal periphery. At the ora serrata, they become absent.

The endothelium of the retina capillaries is non-fenestrated, which prevents large molecules to pass into the retinal tissue (inner blood-retina barrier). The retinal pigment epithelium with its tight junctions also prevents large molecules to pass from the choriocapillaris into the retinal tissue (outer blood-retina barrier). The retinal capillaries have very high-density coverage of pericytes and they lack pre-capillary sphincters, which means that they are continuously perfused. Retinal arterioles, venules, and capillaries are enveloped by microglia cells.

The retinal blood vessels lack autonomic innervations and preserve constant blood flow through autoregulation. Autoregulatory mechanisms (myogenic and metabolic) regulate blood perfusion in the retina during changes in blood pressure, intraocular pressure, and blood gasses. Variations of retinal functional activity (exposure to light, darkness, and flicker stimulation) also activate autoregulatory mechanisms of the retinal blood vessels.

The Vascular System of the Choroid

The choroidal blood vessels are structured in three layers: choriocapillaris (adjacent to Bruch's membrane), Sattler's layer (containing small arterioles/venules), and Haller's layer (containing larger arteries/venules). (Figure 3B) Arterial blood supply derives from the long and short posterior ciliary arteries.

Venous blood outflow from the choroid goes to the four vorticose veins that drain in the superior and inferior ophthalmic veins. Choriocapillaries differ from retinal capillaries: they form many anastomoses, their capillary wall is fenestrated, and there is autonomic (sympathetic and parasympathetic) innervation. The choroidal blood vessels have autoregulatory mechanisms as well, but the response is much weaker than the autoregulation of blood flow in the retina.

The Vascular System of the Ciliary Body and Iris

The iris and ciliary body are supplied by the anterior ciliary arteries, the long posterior ciliary arteries, and anastomotic connections from the anterior choroid. (Figure 4) In the ciliary body, the blood vessels consist of the ciliary arteries, veins, and capillary networks. The capillary endothelium is fenestrated. The major arterial circle is in the ciliary body stroma at the peripheral edge of the iris.

It is formed mainly by the branches of the long posterior ciliary arteries, but also from branches from the anterior ciliary arteries. Radial arteries arise from the major arterial circle and converge in a spinal pattern toward the pupillary margin where they anastomose and form an incomplete – minor arterial circle of the iris. Corresponding veins form the minor venous circle of the iris, but the radiating veins that follow the arteries do not form a major venous circle in the ciliary body. The blood vessels in the iris have autonomic innervation and their capillary endothelium is non-fenestrated.

Discussion

Concerning the fact that ocular circulation is a highly complex system, the methods that aim to evaluate ocular blood flow must be adapted to obtain measurements from the specific ocular vascular bed in order to produce most accurate values. This usually demands highly sophisticated technology and prerequisites about regulation of various external and intrinsic factors that may affect the ocular blood flow. The conditions that have been reported to affect the measurement of ocular blood flow are presented on Table 1.

A protocol should be implemented for each method of measurement and ideally, the standards of the different techniques should implement, where possible, identical conditions of measurement in order to obtain a better correlation of the outcomes from different methods.

Table 1. Factors that affect ocular blood flow

External factors	Systemic factors	Local (ocular) factors
brightness temperature air quality (%O2, %CO2) altitude	body posture exercise age acute and chronic systemic disease blood pressure heart rate blood glucose cholesterol smoking alcohol caffeine systemic medications	intraocular pressure axial length of the globe acute or chronic eye disease topical medication

The importance of accurate evaluation of the various aspects of ocular circulation has three main aspects. The primary aspect is to understand in detail the specifics of the blood vessel physiology in all ocular segments. The second aspect is to be able to monitor the condition of the vascular system in various systemic and ocular pathologies. This is especially relevant in ophthalmic vascular pathology (diabetic retinopathy, hypertensive retinopathy, retinal artery and vein occlusions, etc.), as well as in the ophthalmic conditions that have been associated with abnormal ocular blood flow such as glaucoma, age-related macular degeneration, degenerative myopia, uveitis, etc. The third aspect is the need of accurate investigative methods to study the effect of various therapeutic interventions to the ocular circulation.

The methods of ocular blood flow measurement are many. This chapter introduces the methods that are currently used and their upgraded versions. New emerging techniques of ocular blood flow measurement are also discussed.

Angiography

Fluorescein angiography (FA) and indocyanine-green angiography (ICG) have been used as qualitative methods for analysis of the retinal and choroidal blood flow for about half a century (Agarwal A., 2009). Both standard fundus camera and scanning laser ophthalmoscope (SLO) can be used to obtain FA and ICG. (Figure 5)

In addition to the qualitative analysis, the SLO allows for a quantitative measurement of the blood flow velocity in the retinal vessels (Harris A et al., 2003). The SLO produces laser light beams that are directed to the fundus through a confocal aperture. These laser beams scan the fundus illuminating successive elements of the retina/choroid with very high velocity. The light that is reflected from the fundus is quantified by a photodetector and the output is recorded and displayed in a digital video format. Flow velocity is determined by measuring the transit time of blood between two points on the video monitor that are separated by a known distance. Using SLO, it is possible to measure mean dye velocity in a major retinal artery or vein. Furthermore, by calculating the time that is necessary for the dye to transit from a major artery to a major vein, it is possible to evaluate arteriovenous passage time. Capillary transit velocity is calculated by timing the passage of hypofluorescent particles through perifoveal and epipapillary capillaries, and measuring the distance travelled.

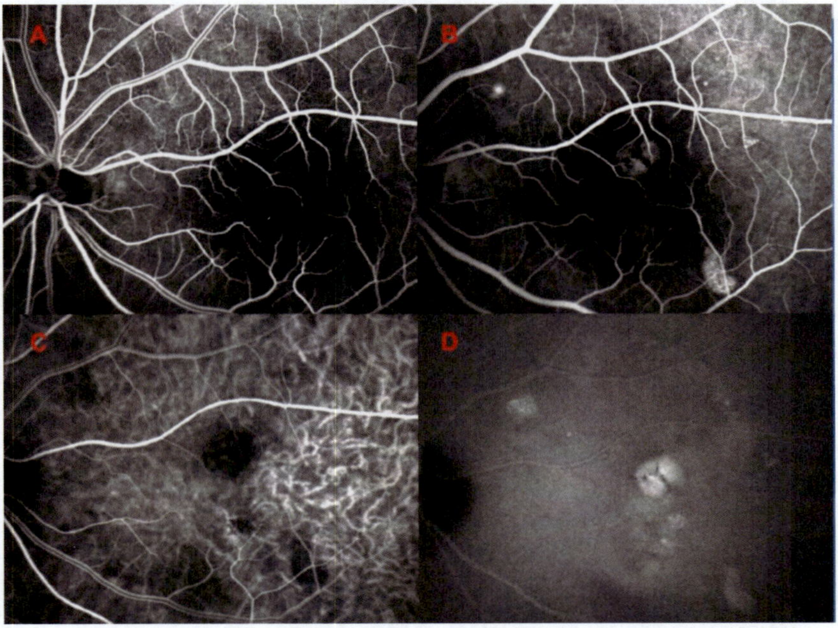

Figure 5. Scanning laser ophthalmoscopy in a case with central serous chorioretinopathy. A. Fluorescein angiography image taken between the first and second minute. B. Fluorescein angiography image taken between the third and fifth minute. C. Indocyanine green angiography image taken before the first minute. D. Indocyanine green angiography image taken between the fifth and fifteenth minute (NIDEK technology).

The recent adaptive optics scanning laser ophthalmoscope (AOSLO) enables direct acquisition of leukocyte movement through the retinal capillaries in the human eye without the use of injected dyes (Martin J.A. and Roorda A., 2009). This device corrects for the optical aberrations of the eye and can take images at high resolution and contrast. The acquisition is being constantly improved by implementing techniques for correction of confounding effects such as the raster scanning and eye and object motion (Tam J. and Roorda A., 2011).

Retinal Function Imager

The retinal function imager is a relatively new technique for qualitative and quantitative analysis of the retinal blood flow (Landa G et al. 2009, Burgansky-Eliash Z. et al. 2012). It comprises of a standard fundus camera, a stroboscopic flash lamp system, and a fast digital camera. The hemoglobin in the erythrocytes is used as a natural chromophore that marks the flow of blood. Blood flow velocity is obtained by measurement of the movement of the erythrocytes inside the blood vessels. This is a noninvasive and convenient method to study the small blood vessels in the retina and to measure the blood flow velocity.

It is also unique in its ability to show circulatory pathways that cannot be seen by other imaging techniques. The limitations of the method is that it must be synchronized with the heartbeat of the patient, the optic media must be clear, the retina that is available for evaluation is the central 35°, and it does not show the non-patent vasculature of the retina.

Retinal Vessel Analyzer

The retinal vessel analyzer is an image analysis unit that computes the data obtained from video images of the retina taken by a conventional fundus camera (Seifert B.U., 2002; Polak K., 2000). The retinal blood vessels that can be measured are to be >90μm diameter. The measurements are taken at a specific cross section of the blood vessels at a distance of approximately 1-2 disc diameters from the optic nerve.

The dynamic vessel analyzer is a retinal vessel analyzer with an addition of visual provocation such as flicker light stimulation and it has been primarily developed for clinical use (Garhofer G., 2010). These devices can measure the retinal vessel diameter as a major determinant of retinal blood flow and vascular resistance. However, they cannot be used for measurement of total volumetric blood flow in the retinal blood vessels, because of the lack of data for blood flow velocity.

Retinal Oximetry

Although retinal oximetry does not estimate ocular blood flow, this method attempts to quantify the major function of the blood circulation, that of oxygenation (Palsson O., 2012).

In order to understand the pathophysiological process of various ocular diseases it is very important to be informed about the level of oxygenation in the blood vessels of the particular condition of interest. Retinal oximetry is a spectrophotometric device that can detect the light absorption of the hemoglobin in the blood. Oxygenated and deoxygenated hemoglobin have different light absorption, therefore by measurement of light absorption of hemoglobin in the retinal blood it is possible to estimate the level of retinal blood oxygenation.

The retinal camera captures images of the fundus at two wavelengths: one is sensitive to the level of hemoglobin oxygen saturation and the other wavelength is similar for both oxygenated and deoxygenated hemoglobin. The image that appears contains color-coded oxygen saturation values and a grayscale retinal image. (Figures 6 and 7) The arterioles are colored in red/orange colors and their saturation normally is 90-100%, while the venules are depicted in blue/green colors and their saturation is usually 50-60%. This method does not provide absolute measurements of oxygenated hemoglobin, and the results are represented in percent.

Using similar methodology as with a fundus camera (optical density ratios), oximetry can also be attained by frequency domain optical coherence tomography (Kagemann L et al., 2007).

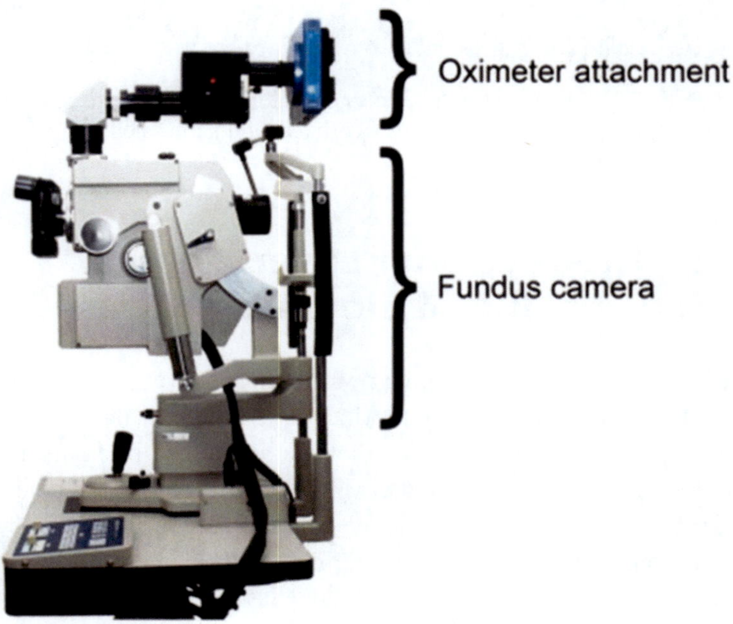

Figure 6. A setting for retinal oxymetry measurement (reprinted with permission from: http://www.oxymap.com/oro.html).

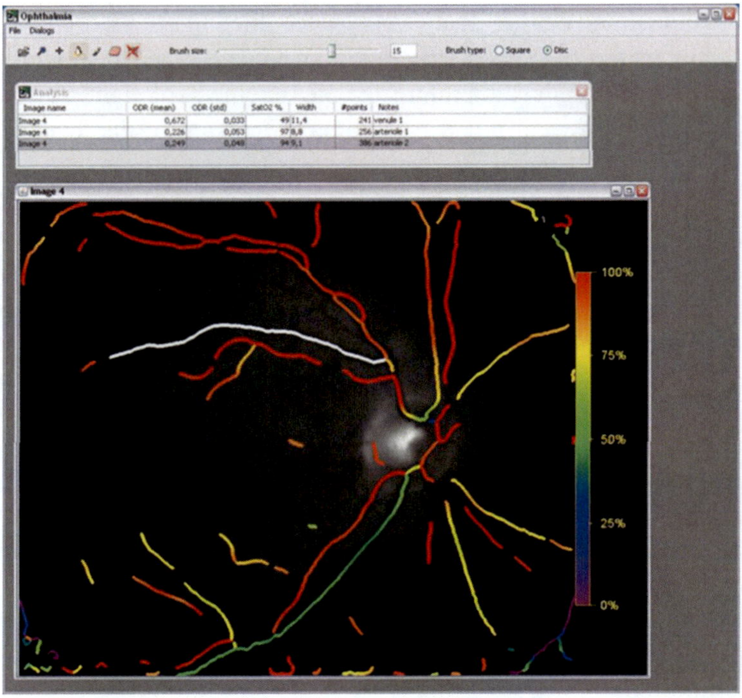

Figure 7. Retinal blood oxymetry - arterioles are colored in red/orange colors and the venules are depicted in blue/green colors (reprinted with permission from: http://www.oxymap.com/oro.html).

Bidirectional Laser Doppler Blood Flowmeter

This is a non-invasive technology that evaluates retinal blood diameter, velocity, and flow. The underlying principle is based on the Doppler effect. Laser light reflected from a moving object is shifted in frequency by an amount that is proportional to the velocity of the moving object. Light scattered from stationary tissue is not shifted and acts as the reference frequency from which a relative change in retinal blood velocity is measured (Feke G.T. and Riva C.E., 1978). A red diode laser is used to measure velocity and a green diode vessel-tracking laser system is used to stabilize and measure the diameter of the vessel of interest. Blood flow is calculated as: ½ x (π/4) x Vmean x 60 x D^2 (Vmean – mean blood velocity, D – vessel diameter). The device is unable to detect the average blood flow velocity, which is calculated from the maximum blood flow velocity. The blood flow parameters are usually acquired from a major retinal artery or vein.

Scanning Laser Doppler Flowmetry

Scanning laser Doppler flowmetry (SLDF) is a method of estimation of retinal tissue blood flow. The infrared laser is directed to a block of tissue (10 μm x 10 μm x 400 μm – 1 pixel) in a retinal area, where the Doppler frequency shifts from moving red blood cells are detected (Harris A. et al., 2003). The SLDF estimates the Doppler frequency shift in each pixel of an area with a size of 2.7×0.7 mm within 2 s. The blood flow parameters detected from the retinal tissue are: velocity, volume, and flow. The data obtained from the SLDF are not influenced only by the tissue hemodynamics, but also by the optical properties of the tissue and by the type of laser light used. Hence, the data is presented in relative units, meaning that SLDF may not be used to compare blood flow data between individuals. This method may be used for prospective studies of blood flow in the same individual and at the same study area or in studies that investigate correlation of blood flow in different vascular beds (Dimitrova et al., 2005). Continuous laser Doppler flowmeter (LDF) (Riva et al., 2010) is an older version of measurement of tissue blood flow. It has been used for evaluation of the blood flow in the iris, the optic nerve head, and the subfoveal choroid. Similar to the SLDF, this method also provides data regarding tissue blood velocity, volume, and flow. However, unlike the SLDF device, the LDF device is not confocal, meaning cell movements from both the superficial and deep tissue layers of the fundus are recorded. Therefore, when evaluating choroidal blood flow, the measurement is taken at the fovea, which is devoid of retinal capillaries and it is assumed at this point only the choroidal blood flow is assessed.

Laser Speckle

Laser speckle is used for quantitative estimation of the microcirculation in the iris, the optic nerve head, the retina, and the choroid (Sugiyama et al., 2010). The laser speckle phenomenon appears when coherent light is directed to a surface, the backscatter of the laser light varies according to the optic properties of the tissue. (Figure 8)

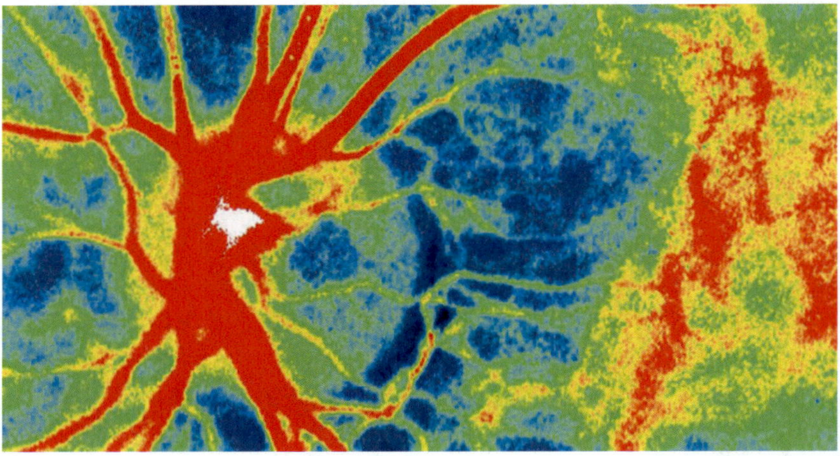

Figure 8. Laser speckle image (courtesy of Prof.Dr. H. Fujii (http://www.softcare-ltd.co.jp/)).

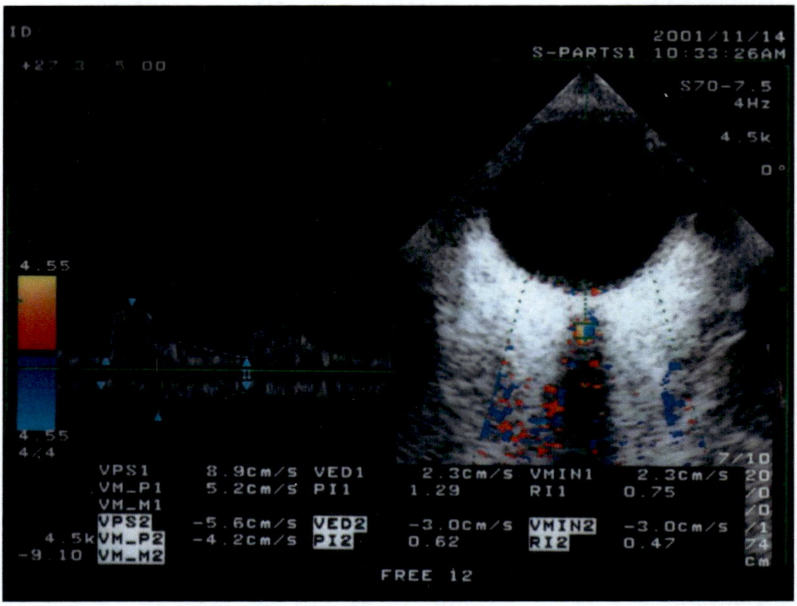

Figure 9. Color Doppler imaging of the central retinal artery and vein. On the left side of the image are velocity waves of the central retinal artery (above the green line) and of the central retinal vein (below the green line). The right side of the image is a B sonography scan with color Doppler imaging of the blood vessels in the retrobulbar area. The ultrasound gate (green vertical line) is positioned at the central retinal artery and vein.

Moving blood cells in the tissue change the backscatter pattern depending on the blood cell velocity. Diode laser can be used to assess microcirculation in the iris, the optic nerve head, and the choroid (in the foveal area). Blue-component argon laser is used for assessment of the retinal microcirculation. Given the fact the laser speckle is affected not only by the movement of the blood cells, but also by the optical properties in the tissue, the measured outcomes are in arbitrary units. Therefore, only studies of the blood flow in the same location of the eye in the same individual at different conditions or at different time intervals is possible. Experimental studies have reported high correlation of the ocular microcirculation assessed by laser speckle with in vivo and in vitro circulatory models (Sugiyama et al., 2010).

Frequency Domain Optical Coherence Tomography

Optical coherence tomography (OCT) has been widely used as an imaging method for ocular tissue analysis in the past decade. This is an interferometric method where light is directed to the ocular structures. The reflected light from the ocular tissue is then registered and processed to depict the ocular tissue layers with a resolution of a few micrometers. Depending on the method of reflected light detection, OCT can be either time-domain (the optical path length of the reference light is translated longitudinally in time) or frequency-domain (acquisition of the interference with spectrally separated detectors). The frequency domain (FD) OCT has a higher imaging speed and improved signal-to-noise ratio than the time domain OCT has. Ultra-high speed FD OCT may detect the Doppler shift of reflected light from moving blood cells in the retinal tissue, which is used to estimate blood flow in the retina (White B.R. et al., 2003). Total venous blood flow of the retina has been measured using Doppler FD OCT by making peripapillary circular scans that transect all the blood vessels in the area (Wang et al., 2009). This method enables volumetric blood flow measurement because it is possible to evaluate both blood flow velocity and blood vessel diameter. The blood flow measurements reported using this method in healthy subjects were within the range of previously published values using laser Doppler flowmetry.

FD-OCT has also been used for evaluating the ocular fundus pulsation, as an indicator of the choroidal pulsatile blood flow (Singh et al., 2011) and for analysis of retinal blood oxygenation (Kagemann et al., 2007).

Color Doppler Imaging

Color Doppler imaging (CDI) may be the most frequently used method for measurement of ocular blood flow parameters (Dimitrova G., and Kato S., 2010, Stalmans I., et al., 2012). It is an ultrasonography device that utilizes the Doppler effect for detection of the velocity of moving blood cells in the vascular system of the eye. (Figure 9)

The blood vessels that are examined by CDI are: the ophthalmic artery and veins, the central retinal artery and vein, posterior ciliary artery and vein, the vortex veins, and the intraocular blood vessels in various ophthalmic pathologies (tumors, retinal detachment, etc.) This method is convenient because it is not invasive and, what is clinically most relevant, it is not dependent on the clarity of the ocular optic media. However, CDI is not sensitive enough for detection of the diameter in most of the retrobulbar blood vessels because of their small size. Therefore, it is not possible to measure volumetric blood flow in those vessels.

The blood flow parameters that can be measured with CDI are: peak systolic (PSV), mean (MV) and end-diastolic (EDV) blood flow velocity, index of resistivity (RI), and index of pulsatility (PI). With regard to the pulsatile character of the venous blood flow in the retrobulbar central retinal vein, the blood flow parameters in this vessel differ because probably they are not under direct influence of the systole and diastole. Therefore, instead of PSV, there is maximum blood velocity (V-max) and instead of EDV, there is minimum blood velocity (V-min) in the central retinal vein. The other blood flow parameters are the same as those in the other blood vessels.

The blood velocity measurements in CDI are dependent on the Doppler angle effect, meaning that the ultrasound wave must be as parallel as possible to the blood vessel being measured. The RI and PI are not dependent on the Doppler angle. Although these indices have been used as markers of vascular damage, they have limited possibility of showing the velocity wave pattern. The blood velocity wave shape can be monitored by the examiner, but until recently, it could not have been quantified. Lockhart et al. (2011) have employed a time-frequency spectral analysis method to quantify changes in the entire velocity flow waveform structure in the ophthalmic and the central retinal artery. They were able to show clear reproducible frequency differences between patients with diabetes type 1 and control subjects, while the RI in both groups was statistically irrelevant. Therefore, time-frequency spectral analysis of CDI may be used to acquire other information that may distinguish between normal and abnormal blood flow characteristics.

Magnetic Resonance Imaging

Magnetic resonance imaging (MRI) is generally regarded as an anatomic imaging technique. However, the constant advancement of the functional MRI technology has given rise to the possibility to use this method for quantification of ocular blood flow. (Maleki N. et al., 2010) Using the arterial spin labeling enables to tag endogenous water in the blood as a marker, without the need to use contrast agent (Zhang et al., 2012). Quantifying ocular blood flow using MRI needs further improvement in spatiotemporal resolution.

Furthermore, being a costly method, it may not be very practical for regular ocular blood flow evaluation. However, it is advantageous over the other methods of ocular blood flow measurement due to its ability to attain quantitative values of total blood flow in ml/min/ml tissue, and because it provides a large field of view without depth limitation. Furthermore, in addition to blood flow measurement, MRI has the potential to attain anatomical aspects, oxygenation, and functional data in the same setting that may prove as a unique clinical and research tool.

Blue-Light Entoptic Phenomenon

This is a method for evaluation of blood flow velocity in the perifoveal retinal capillaries. It involves comparison of the velocity of cells movement on a monitor with the velocity of the leukocytes in the perifoveal capillaries of the subject's eye that has been illuminated with a blue light (wavelength 430 nm) (Fallon et al., 1986). Given its subjective nature, this method is not used often at present.

Infrared Thermography

Infrared thermography is a method that can be used for measurement of ocular surface temperature. Among the factors that influence ocular surface temperature are: external and body temperature, tear film characteristics and ocular blood flow (Kessel L. et al., 2010). Measurement of ocular surface temperature has been used as an indirect indicator of ocular blood flow (Sodi A. et al., 2009).

Although this method does not give direct measurement of the blood flow, it is fast, safe, and non-invasive and may give an overall estimation of the ocular blood flow in various eye conditions. The clinical applicability and significance of infrared thermography for the estimation of ocular blood flow need further evaluation.

Laser Interferometry

Laser interferometry in ophthalmology has been used for evaluating ocular fundus pulsation (Hommer A. et al., 2008). Ocular fundus pulsation is the distance variation between cornea and retina during the cardiac cycle. Because the eye is a closed compartment, during the systole the bulk blood inflow in the eye causes the chorioretina to distend, while during the diastole the blood outflow decreases the volume of the chorioretina.

The distension and diminution of the chorioretinal volume causes variation in the intraocular distance between the retina and cornea. The laser interferometer measures the distance between the retina and the anterior surface of the cornea during systole and diastole. This is achieved by illuminating the eye by a collimated laser beam of long coherence light. Part of the light is reflected at the front of the corneal surface, and another part at the ocular fundus.

The laser interferometer device calculates the differences of the distances between the fundus and corneal surface during systole and diastole. The maximum distance change during the cardiac cycle is called fundus pulsation amplitude (FPA) and it has been used for estimation of choroidal blood flow. This is an indirect method of blood flow measurement that assumes a non-pulsatile venous blood outflow.

In addition, ocular biomechanical properties, such ocular rigidity affect the outcomes. A novel technique had been developed that enables measurement of fundus pulsations at a preselected ocular layer, unlike the previous methods that only enabled reflection from the strongest reflecting retinal layer (Dragostinoff N. et al., 2009).

However, a new custom-designed FD-OCT system was developed that could achieve simultaneous measurement of corneal and retinal positions with high accuracy (Singh K. et al., 2011). By using this method, it was possible to evaluate the pulsatility of the structures of the eye with very high precision, which was superior to laser interferometry.

Pneumotonometry (Pulsatile Ocular Blood Flow)

The pulsatile ocular blood flow is calculated from the temporal variation of intraocular pressure and it is based on a hydrodynamic eye model. Several methods have been used to study the pulsatile component of the ocular blood flow (Hoffmann et al., 2004; Entenmann B. et al., 1997; Langham 1989; Harris et al., 2003). These methods use either a contact lens (Entenmann B. et al., 1997), a tonometry tip (Hoffmann et al., 2004) or air (Harris et al., 2003) in order to make continuous measurements of the intraocular pressure. From those measurements, the mean ocular pressure pulse amplitude is evaluated by calculating the difference between the maximum and minimum intraocular pressure. The pulse amplitude of the intraocular pressure is considered to represent the change in intraocular blood volume during a cardiac cycle. The change of intraocular blood volume has mostly been attributed to the blood volume change in the choroid.

These methods can also be used for ophthalmodynamometry in order to study the blood pressures in the intraocular blood vessels (Entenmann B. et al., 1997). This is achieved using a suction cup placed on the sclera that can gradually increase the intraocular pressure. The examiner observes the fundus while the intraocular pressure is being increased. The pressure is elevated until the examiner observes absence of blood flow in the central retinal artery, which is recorded as systolic blood pressure in the central retinal artery. Then the pressure is being decreased until the observer can see no pulsation in the central retinal artery that is recorded as diastolic blood pressure in the central retinal artery. The methods for pulsatile ocular blood flow measurement are indirect estimations of choroidal blood flow that assume a non-pulsatile intraocular venous outflow. Furthermore, in addition to the ocular blood flow, other factors such as ocular rigidity and corneal thickness may influence the intraocular pressure measurement. With the introduction of dynamic contour tonometer, it is possible to attain the intraocular pressure and ocular pulse amplitude continuously while excluding the effect of the corneal thickness (Hoffmann et al., 2004).

An overview of the methods of ocular blood flow measurement is presented in Table 2. Given the information presented in Table 2, it is possible to conclude that most of the methods used for ocular blood flow measurement are dependent on the clarity of the optic media.

Table 2. Methods of ocular blood flow measurement (Legend: CV – coefficient of variation, SD –standard deviation)

Method of ocular blood flow measurement	Ocular vascular bed	Major circulatory parameters	Invasiveness, use of contrast	Dependence on clarity of optic media	Reproducibility	Direct/ indirect method
Scanning laser ophthalmoscope (Fluorescein angiography)	Branches of intraocular central retinal artery and vein	Mean blood flow velocity, mean arterio-venous passage time	Invasive, use of fluorescein dye	Yes	15%-18% CV	Direct
Scanning laser ophthalmoscope (Indocyanine green angiography)	Choroidal blood vessels in an arbitrary area of interest	Dye dilution curves, rate of dye passage	Invasive, use of indocyanine green dye	Yes	18% CV	Direct
Retinal Function Imager	Intraocular retinal blood vessels	Blood flow velocity	Noninvasive	Yes	7.5% CV	Direct
Retinal vessel analyzer	Intraocular retinal blood vessels	Blood vessel diameter	Noninvasive	Yes	1.3% CV in arteries, 2.6% CV in veins	Direct
Retinal oximetry	Intraocular blood vessels in the retina	Percent of oxygenated hemoglobin	Noninvasive	Yes	1.0% SD in arteries 1.4% SD in veins	Direct
Bidirectional laser Doppler flowmeter	Branches of intraocular central retinal artery and vein	Blood vessel diameter, blood flow velocity, blood flow	Noninvasive	Yes	16%-22% CV	Direct
Scanning Laser Doppler flowmetry	Retinal tissue blood circulation	Blood flow velocity, blood flow volume, tissue blood flow	Noninvasive	Yes	<6% intraobserver reproducibility	Direct
Laser Doppler flowmeter	Iridal, choroidal and optic nerve head tissue blood circulation	Blood flow velocity, blood flow volume, total blood flow	Noninvasive	Yes	<25% CV for choroidal blood flow <32% CV for optic nerve head blood flow	Direct

Method of ocular blood flow measurement	Ocular vascular bed	Major circulatory parameters	Invasiveness, use of contrast	Dependence on clarity of optic media	Reproducibility	Direct/ indirect method
Laser Speckle	Iridal, choroido-retinal, optic nerve head tissue and retinal veins of small diameter	Blood flow velocity	Noninvasive	Yes	<9.7 % CV for choroid-retina <13% CV for optic nerve head 2.5% CV for retinal venules	Direct
Doppler FD-OCT	Branches of intraocular central retinal artery and vein	Blood vessel diameter, blood velocity and flow	Noninvasive	Yes	10.5% CV for retinal vein blood flow	Direct
Color Doppler imaging	Retrobulbar blood vessels (central retinal artery and vein, posterior ciliary arteries, ophthalmic arteries), vortex veins, intraocular tumor vessels, retinal neovascularisation etc.	blood velocity, resistivity and pulsatility indices	Noninvasive	No	4.8% CV for the central retinal artery 38.8% CV for the ophthalmic artery	Direct
Magnetic resonance imaging	Bulk choroido-retinal blood flow	Total blood flow	Noninvasive	No	30% SD	Direct
Blue-light entoptic phenomenon	Perifoveal capillaries	Blood (leukocyte) velocity	Noninvasive	Yes/No	80% repeatability	Direct
Infrared thermography	Bulk ocular blood flow	Corneal temperature	Noninvasive	No	<1.5% SD	Indirect
Laser interferometry	Choroid	Fundus pulsation amplitude	Noninvasive	Yes	4.9% CV	Indirect
Pneumotonometry	Choroid	Intraocular pressure pulsation amplitude, pulsatile ocular blood flow	Noninvasive	No	10.6% CV	Indirect

The measurement methods that are independent of clarity of optic media are color Doppler imaging, functional MRI, pulsatile ocular blood flow methods, and infrared thermography. The majority of the methods are direct measurements of the ocular circulatory characteristics. The indirect methods used for ocular blood flow are infrared thermography, laser interferometry, and pneumotonometry. The parameters that these methods evaluate (corneal temperature, fundus pulsation amplitude, and pressure pulse amplitude) mostly or partially are attributed to the ocular blood flow; however, there are additional factors that affect the results. Reproducibility of the methods is presented either as reproducibility, repeatability, and coefficient of variation, or, as standard deviation, depending on the availability of data. Most of the techniques have acceptable reproducibility. To the best of our knowledge, the highest reproducibility was reported with retinal vessel analyzer and oximetry.

Ocular blood measurement technology is generally quite expensive and institutions that can afford it are usually high standard academic centers. Those methods that are practical and affordable for smaller institutions may be mostly indirect methods for ocular blood flow measurement such as thermography, pneumotonometry, and blue-light entoptoscopy.

Conclusion

An ideal method for ocular blood flow measurement would be safe, noninvasive, accurate, reproducible, specific to the vascular bed that is being evaluated, fast to acquire and analyze data, direct, independent of the optic media clarity, and inexpensive. Presently there is no such method, however, we are witnessing a constant improvement of the existing methods and emergence of new techniques for ocular blood flow measurement. Except for the high cost and the prerequisite of clear optic media, FD OCT may be currently the closest to the ideal method. The advantage of FD OCT is that, in addition to acquiring anatomic status, it can be used to measure total volumetric blood flow, fundus pulsation amplitude, and level of oxygenation at the same setting. On the other hand, clarity of optic media may be most affected in the population where acquisition of blood flow may be of highest necessity – in the aged and diseased eye. Hence, the importance of improvement of techniques that are independent of the presence of optic media opacities.

Most of the techniques that are presented in this chapter evaluate specific characteristics or sites of measurement of the ocular circulation. Although we may suggest an optimal method that may cover most of the relevant aspects of the circulatory status of the eye, the abundance of imaging modalities today enables us to study different aspects of the ocular blood flow.

References

Agarwal A. Fundus fluorescein and indocyanine green angiography: a textbook and atlas. 1st ed. Thorofare: Slack Incorporated, 2008.

Burgansky-Eliash Z., Lowenstein A., Neuderfer M., et al., 2012. The Correlation between Retinal Blood Flow Velocity Measured by the Retinal Function Imager and Various Physiological Parameters. *Ophthalmic Surg Lasers Imaging*. 10:1-8. doi: 10.3928/15428877-20120802-01.

Dimitrova G., Kato S., 2010. Color Doppler imaging of retinal diseases. *Surv. Ophthalmol.* 55(3):193-214.

Dimitrova G, Tomita G and Kato S, 2005. Correlation between capillary blood flow of retina estimated by SLDF and circulatory parameters of retrobulbar blood vessels estimated by CDI in diabetic patients. *Graefe's Arch. Clin. Exp. Ophthalmol.* 243:653-8.

Dragostinoff N., Werkmeister R.M., Gröschl M., et al., 2009. Depth-resolved measurement of ocular fundus pulsations by low-coherence tissue interferometry. *J. Biomed. Opt.* 14(5):054047. doi: 10.1117/1.3251049.

Entenmann B., Robert Y.C., Pirani P., et al., 1997. Contact lens tonometry-application in humans. *Invest. Ophthalmol. Vis. Sci.* 38(12):2447-51.

Fallon T.J., Chowiencyzk P., Kohner E.M., 1986. Measurement of retinal blood flow in diabetes by the blue-light entoptic phenomenon. *Br. J. Ophthalmol.* 70(1):43-6.

Feke G.T. and Riva C.E., 1978. Laser Doppler measurements of blood velocity in human retinal vessels. *J. Opt. Soc. Am.* 68: 526–531.

Garhofer G. Bek T., Boehm A.G., et al., 2010. Use of the retinal vessel analyzer in ocular blood flow research. *Acta Ophthalmol.* 88(7):717-22.

Harris A., Jonescu-Cuypers C.P., Kagemann L., Ciulla T.A., Krieglstein G.K. Atlas of ocular blood flow. 1st ed. Philadelphia: Butterwoth Heinemann, 2003.

Hoffmann E.M., Grus F.H., Pfeiffer N., 2004. Intraocular pressure and ocular pulse amplitude using dynamic contour tonometry and contact lens tonometry. *BMC Ophthalmol.* 23;4:4.

Hommer A., Fuchsjäger-Mayrl G., Resch H., et al., 2008. Estimation of ocular rigidity based on measurement of pulse amplitude using pneumotonometry and fundus pulse using laser interferometry in glaucoma. *Invest. Ophthalmol. Vis. Sci.* 49(9):4046-50.

Kagemann L., Wollstein G., Wojtkowski M., et al., 2007. Spectral oximetry assessed with high-speed ultra-high-resolution optical coherence tomography. *J. Biomed. Opt.* 12(4): 041212. doi: 10.1117/1.2772655

Kessel L., Johnson L., Arvidsson H., et al., 2010. The Relationship between Body and Ambient Temperature and Corneal Temperature. *Invest Ophthalmol Vis. Sci.*.51(12):6593-6597.

Kiel J.W., 2010. The Ocular Circulation. San Rafael (CA): Morgan and Claypool Life Sciences; 2010.

Kur J., Newmana E.A., Chan-Ling T., 2012. Cellular and physiological mechanisms underlying blood flow regulation in the retina and choroid in health and disease. *Progress in Retinal and Eye Research*. 31, 377-406.

Landa G., Garcia P.M., Rosen R.B., 2009. Correlation between retina blood flow velocity assessed by retinal function imager and retina thickness estimated by scanning laser ophthalmoscopy/optical coherence tomography. *Ophthalmologica*.223(3):155-61.

Langham M.E., Farrell R.A., O'Brien V., et al., 1989. Blood flow in the human eye. *Acta Ophthalmol. Suppl.* 191:9-13.

Lockhart C.J., McCann A., Agnew C.A., et al., 2011. Impaired microvascular properties in uncomplicated type 1 diabetes identified by Doppler ultrasound of the ocular circulation. *Diab. Vasc. Dis. Res.* 8(3):211-20.

Maleki N., Dai W., Alsop D.C., 2011. Blood flow quantification of the human retina with MRI. *NMR Biomed.* 24(1):104-11.

Martin J.A., Roorda A., 2009. Pulsatility of parafoveal capillary leukocytes. *Exp. Eye Res*. 88(3):356-60.

Palsson O., Geirsdottir A., Hardarson S.H., et al, 2012. Retinal oximetry images must be standardized: a methodological analysis. *Invest. Ophthalmol. Vis. Sci.* 53(4):1729-33. doi: 10.1167/iovs.11-8621.

Polak K., Dorner G., Kiss B., et al, 2000. Evaluation of the Zeiss retinal vessel analyzer. *Br. J. Ophthalmol.* 84(11):1285-90.

Riva C.E., Geiser M., Petrig B.L., 2010. Ocular blood flow assessment using continuous laser Doppler flowmetry. *Acta Ophthalmol.* 88(6):622-9.

Seifertl B.U., Vilser W., 2002. Retinal Vessel Analyzer (RVA)--design and function. *Biomed. Tech.* 47 Suppl. 1 Pt. 2:678-81.

Singh K., Dion C., Wajszilber M., Ozaki T., et al., 2011. Measurement of ocular fundus pulsation in healthy subjects using a novel Fourier-domain optical coherence tomography. *Invest Ophthalmol Vis Sci.* Nov 21;52(12):8927-32.

Snell R.S., Lemp M.A. Clinical anatomy of the eye. 2nd ed. Malden: Blackwell Science, 1998.

Sodi A., Giambene B., Miranda P., et al., 2009. Ocular surface temperature in diabetic retinopathy: a pilot study by infrared thermography. *Eur. J. Ophthalmol.* 19(6):1004-8.

Stalmans I., Vandewalle E., Anderson D.R., et al, 2012. Use of color Doppler imaging in ocular blood flow research. *Acta Ophthalmol.* 89(8):e609-30.

Sugiyama T., et al., 2010. Use of laser speckle flowgraphy in ocular blood flow research. *Acta Ophthalmol.* 88(7):723-9.

Tam J. and Roorda A., 2011. Speed quantification and tracking of moving objects in adaptive optics scanning laser ophthalmoscopy. *Journal of Biomedical Optics.* 16(3), 036002.

Wang Y., Lu A., Gil-Flamer J., et al., 2009. Measurement of total blood flow in the normal human retina using Doppler Fourier-domain optical coherence tomography. *Br. J. Ophthalmol.* 93(5):634-7.

White B., Pierce M., Nassif N., et al., 2003. In vivo dynamic human retinal blood flow imaging using ultra-high-speed spectral domain optical coherence tomography. *Opt. Express.* 11(25):3490-7.

Zhang Y., San Emeterio Nateras O., Peng Q., et al., 2012. Blood flow MRI of the human retina/choroid during rest and isometric exercise. *Invest. Ophthalmol. Vis. Sci.* 28;53(7):4299-305.

In: Recent Advances in Ophthalmology Research ISBN: 978-1-62808-021-6
Editor: Galina Dimitrova

Chapter 3

Neurodegeneration in Glaucoma and Alzheimer's Disease

***Stanley Park*[1] *and Yvonne Ou*[2,*]**
[1]Ohio State University College of Medicine, Columbus, Ohio, US
[2]University of California, San Francisco, San Francisco, California, US

Abstract

Glaucoma, the leading cause of irreversible blindness worldwide, is a neurodegenerative disorder characterized by stereotyped retinal ganglion cell (RGC) loss with optic nerve cupping and corresponding visual field defects. The disease pathogenesis is not very well understood, but the initial site of injury is thought to the RGC axon as it passes through the pores of the lamina cribrosa at the optic nerve head. Focal axonal injury is likely a key component of RGC glaucomatous pathology, followed by eventual neuronal soma apoptosis and irreversible RGC death. However, our understanding of the pathological cellular processes that occur between initial injury and cell death is still evolving. Emerging evidence supports the hypothesis that the pathological degeneration of a stressed RGC may be compartmentalized at the subcellular level, specifically at the soma, axon, dendrite and synapse. This paradigm is well-recognized in other neurodegenerative diseases, such as Alzheimer disease (AD), in which synapse loss precedes neuronal death and may even correlate to early stages of clinical disease. In this review, we examine some of the

[*] E-mail: OuY@vision.ucsf.edu.

compartmentalized changes that occur in other neurodegenerative diseases such as AD, and how these changes may play a role in glaucomatous neurodegeneration.

Keywords: Glaucoma, Alzheimer disease, compartmentalized neuro-degeneration, synaptic, dendritic, and axonal degeneration

Introduction

Glaucoma is a neurodegenerative disease that causes irreversible blindness. It is characterized by progressive optic nerve head cupping, retinal nerve fiber layer thinning, and eventually, retinal ganglion cell (RGC) death. Glaucoma is the leading cause of irreversible blindness worldwide and disproportionately affects females and Asians. [1, 2] Moreover, it is the leading cause of blindness among African Americans. [2-4] Lowering intraocular pressure (IOP), the only modifiable risk factor in glaucoma, can be insufficient for some patients as disease progression is evident despite reasonable IOP. [5-7] What makes glaucoma difficult to treat is that it is estimated that approximately 50% of glaucoma patients are unaware of their disease. [3] To add to this, ophthalmologists are currently underequipped to detect glaucoma early in the clinic. It is estimated that 25-35% of RGCs are lost before statistically abnormal changes are seen on automated visual field tests. [8] In this chapter, we will review a growing body of evidence that supports the idea of compartmentalized degeneration of RGCs. Discovering earlier disease markers and novel therapeutic targets at multiple subcellular compartments will likely be necessary to adequately subdue disease progression.

Alzheimer Disease (AD) is the most common cause of dementia. It, too, is a neurodegenerative disease and is characterized by cerebral proteopathy. For definitive diagnosis in a patient, it requires the presence of clinical dementia to the extent that impairs daily activities, as well as pathologic intracellular neurofibrillary tangles (NFTs) made of hyperphosphorylated tau and extracellular amyloid beta (Aβ) plaques. The gross pathology of AD comprises atrophy of the hippocampus and cortex. [9-11] An ageing population and a lack of disease modifying treatments will increase AD cases beyond 100 million people by 2050 in the United States with an estimated care cost of 1 trillion dollars.[12, 13] For health care systems to shoulder this rising burden, it is prudent for physicians and scientists to improve methods of treatment.

Like glaucoma, difficulty managing AD is likely due to multifactorial insults to neuronal compartments, some of which are affected by amyloid and tau.

Glaucoma and AD are thought to share, at least in part, some commonalities as both are age-related neurodegenerative diseases. The link between the two diseases was first observed in 1978, when Chandra and colleagues noted a higher frequency of glaucoma in patients with AD through a retrospective analysis of death certificates.[14] Bayer and colleagues supported this finding in 2002 when they investigated the prevalence of glaucoma in a group of institutionalized patients in Germany by comparing patients who had AD to those who did not. Strikingly, 24.5% of patients with AD had glaucoma compared to 6.5% in the control group. 100% of patients with AD and glaucoma were normotensive (defined as IOP less than 23 mmHg) which suggests that AD patients may have RGCs that are more vulnerable to IOP.[15] Similarly when Tamura and colleagues compared Japanese patients with AD to matched non-AD controls, 23.8% of AD patients also had glaucoma while 9.9% of the control group had glaucoma.[16] On the other hand, it appears that patients with glaucoma are not at increased risk of developing AD. In a large retrospective analysis of 11,721 patients with primary open angle glaucoma, Kessing and colleagues did not find that these patients had increased risk of developing AD.[17] In another study, Bach-Holm and colleagues found that 69 normal tension glaucoma patients did not develop AD over twenty years.[16] More recently, the largest study on the prevalence of AD in open-angle glaucoma patients using 5% Medicare claims data demonstrated that patients with a diagnosis of glaucoma had a lower rate of AD diagnosis compared to patients without glaucoma (6% reduced hazard).[18] However, this study did not account for disease severity, and it is therefore possible that more advanced cases of glaucoma and AD are related.

These studies show a higher prevalence of glaucoma in patients with AD while other studies fail to show evidence for the reverse. Bayer and colleagues showed that patients having both AD and glaucoma exhibit an accelerated rate of visual field decline.[19] In support of this, optical coherence tomography (OCT) enabled the first demonstration of structural defects analogous to glaucoma in AD patients. In this study, the nerve fiber layer thickness was found to be significantly thinner in 17 AD patients when compared to 14 age-matched normal controls.[20] Interestingly, postmortem studies show that visual defects found in AD patients are likely early signs of disease. McKee and colleagues found Aβ and NFTs in Visual Association-Brodman 19 of patients who had no clinical cognitive impairment.[21] Some brains displayed an absence of pathology in usual hippocampal and cortical areas, an indication that AD's onset may quietly begin at the visual centers and undergo retrograde degeneration of the visual pathway ultimately killing the RGC. Other groups support this by reporting AD-associated proteopathy near atrophied lateral geniculate ganglia.[22, 23]

Clinical studies supporting the association between glaucoma and AD naturally led to a discussion regarding a possible common molecular pathophysiology. The planarity that appears to exist in a neuron's response to localized insults is an exciting prospect for unifying our collective understanding of neurodegenerative diseases. It is likely that many neurodegenerative diseases have overlapping pathophysiological mechanisms. Glaucoma and AD could share similar therapeutic obstacles because of the potentially overlapping pathways observed in different compartments of the afflicted neurons. In this review chapter we explore this possible paradigm in the context of the axon, dendrite, and synapse. We outline the current understanding of each compartment's potential contribution to these two diseases in hopes that a better understanding of these processes can lead to improvement of detection and treatment.

Synapse and Dendrite Pathology

There is a growing body of work that supports the hypothesis that it is synaptic and dendritic pathology, not the presence of visible amyloid plaques or NFTs, which strongly correlates with the clinical symptoms of AD.[24-26] Immunohistochemistry of postmortem AD tissue display loss of synaptic proteins such as synaptophysin while exhibiting sparse synaptic density and concomitantly enlarged presynaptic components.[24, 27, 28] The postsynaptic compartments, namely the stubby and mushroom dendritic spines, are smaller, fewer in number and are replaced by aberrant ones. In the last few decades, the pathological and genetic hallmarks of AD have been studied to elucidate the mechanism for these observed synaptic and dendritic aberrations. In this section we discuss how soluble oligomer amyloid beta (oAβ) and NFTs contribute to synapse and dendrite pathology in AD.

Aβ's physiologic role involves synaptoplasticity and neuronal survival, both canonical elements of memory formation.[29-31] However, in the context of disease it accumulates to toxic levels rising from picomolar to nanomolar concentrations. This accumulation is likely due to mutations or duplications altering amyloid precursor protein (APP) or the presence of the ApoE4 allele. Evidence for oAβ-induced synaptopathology stems from studies done on AD mouse models.[32-37] Using an AD mouse moudel, Spires and colleagues found that there was a 50% decreased dendritic spine density in areas containing amyloid plaques. Interestingly, there was a significant amount of decreased spine density that was not spatially associated with the plaques. To explain this finding, others found that soluble oAβ, not amyloid plaques, is the responsible APP byproduct that results in synaptic and dendritic insults, whereas plaques are a sign of a late and more severe stage of disease.[32, 35, 37, 38]

oAβ damages the synapse through a few possible mechanisms. Studies on the postsynaptic compartment show that oAβs are capable of inducing pores that transmit calcium ions at the synapse altering synaptic transmission.[39, 40]. Another possibility is the induction of receptor clustering whereby glutaminergic receptors aggregate in the synapses leading to excitotoxicity. For example, studies show that oAβ binds and activates receptors like N-methyl-D-aspartate receptors (NMDA-R) and GluR5 to cause subsequent calcium influx resulting in long term depression (LTD) and spine loss.[41-43] Interestingly, oAβ also impairs synaptic transmission to cause LTD. It is implicated in directly binding alpha-amino-3-hydroxy-5-methyl-4-isoxazolepropionic acid receptor (AMPA-R) and NMDA-R to induce receptor internalization.[44] Supporting evidence shows that at the presynaptic terminal, oAβ hinders P/Q calcium currents that also impair synaptic transmission.[45] Further research in oAβ and its action on the synapse may reveal the pathological interplay of excitotoxicity and transmission impairment that eventually leads to LTD and cognitive impairment.

oAβ-associated synapse pathology is compounded by potential contributions from tauopathy. Tau protein is classically known as a microtubule binding protein localized to the axon.[46] Under pathologic conditions, tau becomes hyperphosphorylated by glycogen synthase kinase (GSK3) and aggregates to form intracellular NFTs, impairing several neuronal functions.[46-49] How does tau actually harm synaptic transmission? Hoover and colleagues show that before tau aggregates to form NFTs, phosphorylated tau mislocalizes from the axon to intact dendritic spines early in the disease course. Once there, they appear to impair glutamate receptor trafficking and synaptic anchoring.[50] In addition, tau may play a role in modulating the postsynaptic density namely through Fyn, a local tyrosine kinase. Fyn, under the influence of tau, ramps up NMDA-R action by phosphorylating its GluN2B subunit, worsening excitotoxicity.[51-53] Not unlike oAβ, it is the soluble form of tau that appears to disrupt synaptic plasticity early in the disease course, prior to advanced neurodegeneration.

At the molecular level, the role of Aβ and tau in glaucoma is not well understood. Nonetheless, a striking clinical correlate of the two diseases was seen in the discovery of Aβ and tau in the vitreous of patients with glaucoma which were identical to those found in the CSF of AD patients.[54] In glaucoma models, McKinnon and colleagues showed that APP undergoes abnormal cleavage by caspase 3 leading to the formation of the same harmful oAβ products found in AD.[55, 56] Building on this, Guo and colleagues showed that Aβ accumulated exclusively near the RGC layer. They showed that targeting Aβ formation with antibodies, β-secretase inhibitors, or anti-Aβ aggregators in their model significantly prevented RGC apoptosis by detection of apoptosing retinal cells (DARC) real-time imaging. Interestingly, combination therapy against Aβ proved to be better than monotherapy supporting the idea that attenuating Aβ can be neuroprotective for RGCs.[57] Thus it is possible that the cleaved product of APP by caspase 3 is neurotoxic and contributes to RGC death. The slow accumulation of cleaved APP is a possible explanation for the protracted course of RGC apoptosis as a certain buildup is required before triggering this pathway.[55] Abnormal tau has been reported in the horizontal retinal cells of human glaucoma eyes.[58] The precise mechanism by which these AD-like events occur in glaucoma is not known. However, caspase 3 activation may be a result of a long standing axonal dying back mechanism mediated by the activation of calcium dependent proteases. Therefore, the cleavage of APP by caspase 3 may be a secondary or tertiary event that is a late manifestation of disease.

The finding that dendritic spine loss is evident in postmortem studies of AD patients has been confirmed in human AD hippocampus tissue, which exhibits abnormal dendritic morphology and loss of spines.[37] Evidence suggests that the dendrite pathology in AD appears to be a direct extension of post-synaptic pathology. *In vitro* studies by Shankar and colleagues demonstrated that pyramidal neurons in rat organotypic slices treated with soluble Aβ reduced the number and strength of excitatory synapses by partially inhibiting NMDA-R signaling and attenuating calcium influx into dendritic spines.[59]

Additional support comes from the work done by Hsieh and colleagues, who found that oAβ-induced NMDA-R and AMPA-R internalization was necessary and sufficient to decrease NMDA-mediated signal transmission and spine density.[44] These examples demonstrate that dendrite pathology in AD is likely an extension of Aβ-induced post-synaptic disturbances in homeostasis.

Studies regarding synapse pathology in glaucoma are relatively scarce. What is known so far is that synaptic degeneration may be present in glaucoma animal models. Using a rat ocular hypertension model, Fu and colleagues postulated that there was synaptic disconnection by demonstrating downregulation of c-fos, a marker for neuronal connectivity.[60] Also, NMDA-Rs appear to exhibit compensatory upregulation at the postsynaptic terminal in a glaucoma rodent model. This may be indicative of depletion of pre-synaptic elements through mechanisms that will be discussed in the axonopathy section of this chapter.[61]

Interestingly, another recent study by Crish and colleagues has shown that transport deficits precede signs of synaptic dysfunction. These data may point to synaptic pathology in glaucoma as a secondary phenomenon to an axonal transport defect.[62] Alternatively, glaucoma synaptic pathology has also been studied in the context of the complement factor cascade. Molecular evidence to explain these observations across multiple glaucoma models appear to be due to glial activation and their inappropriate implementation of the complement cascade.[63-67]

The synaptic and dendritic compartments undergo two well known complement-related mechanisms: phagocytosis by recruited microglia and destruction by the membrane attack complex. Astrocyte release of C1q leads to C3 activation. Both proteins opsonize the synaptic area in the inner plexiform layer.[68] In this study it is important to note that the complement factors were upregulated even before there was any visible reduction in synaptic density and much less RGC death.

Dendritic pathology is also found in glaucoma models. In a primate model, there again appears to be thinning, blebbing, and reduced complexity of dendrites that correlates with a reduction in response to visual stimuli.[69, 70] Analogous findings have been published in rat and cat models of glaucoma. [71, 72]

Just as in AD, these findings appear to be an early marker for damage as studies show that these events occur before the RGC soma begins to shrink, even before axon thinning. Still further, not only are the RGC dendrites undergoing changes, the primate models show that there is dendritic atrophy of the LGN, the site to which the RGC axons project.[73] It appears that studies in dendrite pathology in glaucoma are largely descriptive though in other contexts it appears to be independent of cell body apoptosis and possibly linked to the ubiquitin proteasome system (UPS).[74, 75] Advancing our understanding of synapse and dendrite pathology in glaucoma by drawing from AD research may spur forward the identification of disease markers and pathologic mechanisms.

Axon Pathology

Healthy neurons utilize slow and fast axonal transport. Kinesin is an anterograde motor protein that is responsible for carrying membrane organelles such as mitochondria, synaptic vesicle precursors, and other secretory products.[76, 77] Thus axonopathy can be defined as the inability of a neuron to transport cargo between the soma and axon terminal. It results in abnormal axonal morphology and synaptic dysfunction secondary to accumulation of membrane bound organelles, filaments and trophic factors necessary for the maintenance of the distal and proximal components of the neuron.[78-81] Thus axonopathy can occur as a result of either traumatic disruption of the axon membrane or due to pathologic accumulation of protein due to vesicle transport defects.

In AD, axons follow the slow and chronic dying back pattern of degeneration, which, as previously mentioned, is characterized by pathological accumulation of membrane bound organelles that appear as swellings and spheroids on histology.[82] Animal models employing various human APP, tau and presenilin mutations show similar phenotypes.[83] At the molecular level, these cardinal elements of AD appear to be as harmful to the axon as they are to the synapse and dendrite. One molecular mechanism is characterized by aberrations in phosphotransferase pathways. oAβs appear to impair fast axonal transport by abnormally activating kinases such as casein kinase 2 (CK2) and glycogen synthase kinase (GSK3). These activated kinases in turn phosphorylate kinesin's light chain causing bound cargo to dissociate.[84-86] Interestingly, impaired axon transport begins relatively early, before the formation of visible aggregates. For example, mitochondrial transport is acutely impaired by oAβ without the formation of abnormal ultrastructural changes.[87] Similar to oAβ, tau undergoes hyperphosphorylation to activate protein phosphatase 1 (PP1) which activates GSK3 and feeds into the pathway that phosphorylates kinesin's light chain.[88] GSK3 can renew this cycle by hyperphosphorylating more tau.[89] Interestingly, tau may be indirectly involved in its own hyperphosphorylation. Kanaan and colleagues' studies on the squid axon showed that an N-terminal phosphatase activating domain (PAD), a site responsible for facilitating PP1-associated GSK3 phosphorylation, is exposed in various forms of tau.[90] PS1 contains a cytoplasmic domain that can bind GSK3 leading to its activation and subsequent kinesin light chain phosphorylation.[91, 92] With uncontrolled phosphorylation by a ubiquitous kinase such as GSK from many individual sources, treatment of AD at the axon may require the development of specific and localized inhibitors. In addition, targeting the individual culprits may be complicated as partial inhibition of one may result in incomplete containment.

In addition to causing aberrant phosphotransferase pathways leading to impaired cargo transport, AD proteopathy also induces axonal degeneration in a caspase-independent manner through calcium disequilibrium. Song and colleagues showed in an *in vitro* system that Aβ sufficiently causes axonal degeneration in a caspase-independent manner. Second, Aβ itself causes caspase activation that induces cell body apoptosis. Third, Aβ mediated axonal degeneration and subsequent cell body apoptosis is halted by application of a calpain inhibitor calpastatin.[93] Calpain is a calcium dependent protease that has been implicated in axonal degeneration in injury and neurodegeneration models.[94] It is capable of acting on numerous substrates including cytoskeletal proteins and receptors. Taking these three points together, one can envision Aβ somehow inducing pathologic calcium levels distal to the cell body and activating calpain. As dying back axonal degeneration continues with calpain cleaving cytoskeletal elements of the axon, it could eventually activate caspases once the axon regresses close enough to the cell body and induce apoptosis.[94]

Compartmentalized destruction of the axon in glaucoma is hypothesized to be due to vulnerable RGC axons as they come together and dive into the optic nerve passing through the lamina cribrosa (LC).[95] The initial site of the insult is theorized to be at the LC directly due to elevated IOP or secondarily to pressure affecting local astrocyte activation and vascular ischemia.[96-98] Howell and colleagues used the DBA/2J mice to locate the site of early axonal damage.[96] They showed swollen and disorganized axons with increasing severity from the nerve fiber layer to the glial lamina, the murine equivalent of the LC. This was correlated to axonal loss in the lamina that corresponded to sectorial RGC loss in the retina. Next, to prove that the site of said axonal damage in the glial lamina is the actual site of the initial insult, the group used the BAX deficient DBA/2J mice in conjunction with a neurofilament label to show where axons stopped fluorescing. Based on the hypothesis of Wallerian degeneration, the extent of axon survival should be up to the site of initial injury. Indeed, their results showed neurofilament staining halting at the anterior edge of the glial lamina.

The molecular mechanism for axonal degeneration in glaucoma appears to be independent of the pro-apoptotic BCL proteins like Bax and once again due to calcium dysregulation. This echos to some extent how Aβ-mediated axonal degeneration is independent of caspases as caspase activation is a well-established endpoint of pro-apoptotic BCL proteins. Libby and colleagues provided compelling evidence for the existence of spatially unique triggers of destruction in the Bax deficient DBA/2J murine glaucoma model. Bax deficiency rescued the RGC cell body but not the axon, suggesting that axonal degeneration is a mechanistically and temporally distinct process from cell body apoptosis.[99]

To investigate calcium as possibly the responsible inciting mechanism of axonopathy in glaucoma, we begin by looking at an acute crush injury model. In a rat model of optic nerve crush injury, acute axonal degeneration resulted in extracellular calcium influx. Application of calcium channel blockers immediately after the insult blocked the rise in intracellular calcium and nearly stopped axonal degeneration.[100] One of the early ultrastructural changes noted is microtubular proteolysis which likely leads to impaired transport as evidenced by localized axonal blebs and swelling.[100] This is likely the work of calcium dependent proteases such as calpain. To complement this, there appears to be a calcium dependent activation of the UPS pathway. [101] We discussed this pathway's involvement in glaucoma dendrite pathology above; it may be a broad system set into motion to facilitate the degeneration of all neuronal extensions.[102] Yet another way calcium may contribute to glaucoma and even AD-associated axonopathy is its role in promoting oxidative stress. Calcium is capable of producing reactive oxygen species (ROS) by activating nitric oxide synthase (NOS) and nicotinamide adenine dinucleotide phosphate (NADPH) oxidase.[103] ROS are well known to damage the bilipid layers and the integrity of the mitochondria and they may even exacerbate calcium toxicity by releasing intracellular stores.[104, 105] Mouse glaucoma models support the possibility that oxidative stress is involved as evidenced by elevated levels of ceruloplasmin.[106] The aqueous humor of glaucoma patients show elevated levels of anti-oxidative stress markers.[107]

To bring this story of calcium dysregulation closer to a glaucoma model paradigm, an interesting *in vitro* transient axonal stretch model also showed acute and persistent calcium levels in axons with pathological alterations in the cytoskeleton.[108] Staal and colleagues used a glass micropipette to channel a pulse of media over an axon bundle to produce axonal strain but not axotomy. In support of this, a recent study has shown that a calcium receptor called

TRPV1 is upregulated in the setting of applied hydrostatic pressure.[109] Work in other glaucoma models has shown differential defects in axonal transport with anterograde transport being affected before retrograde transport and axonal defects occurring at parts distal to the LC.[62, 110] So rather than elevated IOP producing an all-or-none destruction of the axon at the LC, one can imagine a more subtle and protracted insult involving calcium dysregulation.

Conclusion

Not all glaucoma patients respond to interventions that lower IOP. For others, having a high IOP does not necessarily result in glaucoma.[7] Clearly, there are properties of the RGC that make some more susceptible to IOP than others, and the concept of compartmentalized pathology provides a framework for advancing our understanding of glaucoma. Working within this framework has primed glaucoma research to benefit from discoveries found in other age-related neurodegenerative diseases. As described in the beginning of the chapter, the clinical correlation between glaucoma and AD has been known for a long time, but only recently has molecular evidence revealed a pattern in pathophysiology to support this relationship.

For the RGC in glaucoma, it is tempting to say that impaired axonal transportation leads to the depletion of presynaptic elements such as vesicles that store neurotransmitters and other peptides. This may be an indolent and temporarily reversible insult that eventually leads to permanent structural degeneration. Prolonged calcium elevation may be an early culprit as it is inducible by mechanical pressure. The dysregulation of calcium homeostasis, the activation of the ubiquitin proteasome system resulting in axon degeneration, and the accumulation of reactive oxygen species are all detrimental processes initially compartmentalized outside of the cell body. It may be that only after sufficient dying back degeneration does it give way to cell body apoptosis. Thus, therapies that preserve the structure and function of RGC synapses, dendrites, and axons may preserve visual function and ultimately prevent RGC apoptosis. It is possible that patients may be experiencing subclinical RGC degeneration, thus preserving RGC compartments may significantly delay the progression of disease and preserve vision.

References

[1] Visual Impairment and Blindness Fact Sheet No282. World Health Organization; 2012; Available from: http://www.who.int/mediacentre/factsheets/fs282/en/.

[2] Quigley HA, Broman AT. The number of people with glaucoma worldwide in 2010 and 2020. *The British journal of ophthalmology*. 2006;90(3):262-7. Epub 2006/02/21.

[3] Sommer A, Tielsch JM, Katz J, Quigley HA, Gottsch JD, Javitt J, et al. Relationship between intraocular pressure and primary open angle glaucoma among white and black Americans. The Baltimore Eye Survey. *Archives of ophthalmology*. 1991;109(8):1090-5. Epub 1991/08/01.

[4] Leske MC, Connell AM, Wu SY, Hyman LG, Schachat AP. Risk factors for open-angle glaucoma. The Barbados Eye Study. *Archives of ophthalmology*. 1995;113(7):918-24. Epub 1995/07/01.

[5] The effectiveness of intraocular pressure reduction in the treatment of normal-tension glaucoma. Collaborative Normal-Tension Glaucoma Study Group. *American journal of ophthalmology*. 1998;126(4):498-505. Epub 1998/10/21.

[6] Gordon MO, Beiser JA, Brandt JD, Heuer DK, Higginbotham EJ, Johnson CA, et al. The Ocular Hypertension Treatment Study: baseline factors that predict the onset of primary open-angle glaucoma. *Archives of ophthalmology*. 2002;120(6):714-20; discussion 829-30. Epub 2002/06/07.

[7] Kass MA, Heuer DK, Higginbotham EJ, Johnson CA, Keltner JL, Miller JP, et al. The Ocular Hypertension Treatment Study: a randomized trial determines that topical ocular hypotensive medication delays or prevents the onset of primary open-angle glaucoma. *Archives of ophthalmology*. 2002;120(6):701-13; discussion 829-30. Epub 2002/06/07.

[8] Kerrigan-Baumrind LA, Quigley HA, Pease ME, Kerrigan DF, Mitchell RS. Number of ganglion cells in glaucoma eyes compared with threshold visual field tests in the same persons. *Investigative ophthalmology and visual science*. 2000;41(3):741-8. Epub 2000/03/11.

[9] Consensus recommendations for the postmortem diagnosis of Alzheimer's disease. The National Institute on Aging, and Reagan Institute Working Group on Diagnostic Criteria for the Neuropathological Assessment of Alzheimer's Disease. *Neurobiology of aging*. 1997;18(4 Suppl):S1-2. Epub 1997/07/01.

[10] Braak H, Braak E, Bohl J. Staging of Alzheimer-related cortical destruction. *European neurology*. 1993;33(6):403-8. Epub 1993/01/01.

[11] Mirra SS, Heyman A, McKeel D, Sumi SM, Crain BJ, Brownlee LM, et al. The Consortium to Establish a Registry for Alzheimer's Disease (CERAD). Part II. Standardization of the neuropathologic assessment of Alzheimer's disease. *Neurology*. 1991;41(4):479-86. Epub 1991/04/01.

[12] Wimo A, Prince M. *World Alzheimer Report 2010: The Global Economic Impact of Dementia* (London: Alzheimer's Disease International). 2010:1–56.

[13] Okie S. Confronting Alzheimer's disease. *The New England journal of medicine*. 2011;365(12):1069-72. Epub 2011/10/14.

[14] Chandra V, Bharucha NE, Schoenberg BS. Conditions associated with Alzheimer's disease at death: case-control study. *Neurology*. 1986;36(2):209-11. Epub 1986/02/01.

[15] Bayer AU, Ferrari F, Erb C. High occurrence rate of glaucoma among patients with Alzheimer's disease. *European neurology*. 2002;47(3):165-8. Epub 2002/03/27.

[16] Tamura H, Kawakami H, Kanamoto T, Kato T, Yokoyama T, Sasaki K, et al. High frequency of open-angle glaucoma in Japanese patients with Alzheimer's disease. *Journal of the neurological sciences*. 2006;246(1-2):79-83. Epub 2006/03/28.

[17] Kessing LV, Lopez AG, Andersen PK, Kessing SV. No increased risk of developing Alzheimer disease in patients with glaucoma. *Journal of glaucoma*. 2007;16(1):47-51. Epub 2007/01/17.

[18] Ou Y, Grossman DS, Lee PP, Sloan FA. Glaucoma, Alzheimer disease and other dementia: a longitudinal analysis. *Ophthalmic epidemiology*. 2012;19(5):285-92. Epub 2012/09/18.

[19] Bayer AU, Ferrari F. Severe progression of glaucomatous optic neuropathy in patients with Alzheimer's disease. *Eye* (Lond). 2002;16(2):209-12. Epub 2002/05/04.

[20] Parisi V, Restuccia R, Fattapposta F, Mina C, Bucci MG, Pierelli F. Morphological and functional retinal impairment in Alzheimer's disease patients. *Clinical neurophysiology : official journal of the International Federation of Clinical Neurophysiology*. 2001;112(10):1860-7. Epub 2001/10/12.

[21] McKee AC, Au R, Cabral HJ, Kowall NW, Seshadri S, Kubilus CA, et al. Visual association pathology in preclinical Alzheimer disease. *Journal of neuropathology and experimental neurology*. 2006;65(6):621-30. Epub 2006/06/20.

[22] Leuba G, Saini K. Pathology of subcortical visual centres in relation to cortical degeneration in Alzheimer's disease. *Neuropathology and applied neurobiology*. 1995;21(5):410-22. Epub 1995/10/01.

[23] Armstrong RA. Visual field defects in Alzheimer's disease patients may reflect differential pathology in the primary visual cortex. *Optometry and vision science : official publication of the American Academy of Optometry*. 1996;73(11):677-82. Epub 1996/11/01.

[24] Masliah E, Terry R. The role of synaptic proteins in the pathogenesis of disorders of the central nervous system. *Brain Pathol*. 1993;3(1):77-85. Epub 1993/01/01.

[25] Terry RD, Masliah E, Salmon DP, Butters N, DeTeresa R, Hill R, et al. Physical basis of cognitive alterations in Alzheimer's disease: synapse loss is the major correlate of cognitive impairment. *Annals of neurology*. 1991;30(4):572-80. Epub 1991/10/01.

[26] Scheff SW, DeKosky ST, Price DA. Quantitative assessment of cortical synaptic density in Alzheimer's disease. *Neurobiology of aging*. 1990;11(1):29-37. Epub 1990/01/01.

[27] Masliah E, Terry RD, DeTeresa RM, Hansen LA. Immunohistochemical quantification of the synapse-related protein synaptophysin in Alzheimer disease. *Neuroscience letters*. 1989;103(2):234-9. Epub 1989/08/28.

[28] DeKosky ST, Scheff SW. Synapse loss in frontal cortex biopsies in Alzheimer's disease: correlation with cognitive severity. Annals of neurology. 1990;27(5):457-64. Epub 1990/05/01.

[29] Ramsden M, Henderson Z, Pearson HA. Modulation of Ca2+ channel currents in primary cultures of rat cortical neurones by amyloid beta protein (1-40) is dependent on solubility status. *Brain research*. 2002;956(2):254-61. Epub 2002/11/26.

[30] Plant LD, Boyle JP, Smith IF, Peers C, Pearson HA. The production of amyloid beta peptide is a critical requirement for the viability of central neurons. *The Journal of neuroscience : the official journal of the Society for Neuroscience*. 2003;23(13):5531-5. Epub 2003/07/05.

[31] Reinhard C, Hebert SS, De Strooper B. The amyloid-beta precursor protein: integrating structure with biological function. *The EMBO journal*. 2005;24(23):3996-4006. Epub 2005/10/28.

[32] Spires TL, Meyer-Luehmann M, Stern EA, McLean PJ, Skoch J, Nguyen PT, et al. Dendritic spine abnormalities in amyloid precursor protein transgenic mice demonstrated by gene transfer and intravital multiphoton microscopy. *The Journal of neuroscience : the official*

journal of the Society for Neuroscience. 2005;25(31):7278-87. Epub 2005/08/05.

[33] Games D, Adams D, Alessandrini R, Barbour R, Berthelette P, Blackwell C, et al. Alzheimer-type neuropathology in transgenic mice overexpressing V717F beta-amyloid precursor protein. *Nature*. 1995;373(6514):523-7. Epub 1995/02/09.

[34] Hsiao K, Chapman P, Nilsen S, Eckman C, Harigaya Y, Younkin S, et al. Correlative memory deficits, Abeta elevation, and amyloid plaques in transgenic mice. *Science*. 1996;274(5284):99-102. Epub 1996/10/04.

[35] Mucke L, Masliah E, Yu GQ, Mallory M, Rockenstein EM, Tatsuno G, et al. High-level neuronal expression of abeta 1-42 in wild-type human amyloid protein precursor transgenic mice: synaptotoxicity without plaque formation. *The Journal of neuroscience : the official journal of the Society for Neuroscience*. 2000;20(11):4050-8. Epub 2000/05/20.

[36] Tsai J, Grutzendler J, Duff K, Gan WB. Fibrillar amyloid deposition leads to local synaptic abnormalities and breakage of neuronal branches. *Nature neuroscience*. 2004;7(11):1181-3. Epub 2004/10/12.

[37] Moolman DL, Vitolo OV, Vonsattel JP, Shelanski ML. Dendrite and dendritic spine alterations in Alzheimer models. *Journal of neurocytology*. 2004;33(3):377-87. Epub 2004/10/12.

[38] Spires-Jones TL, Meyer-Luehmann M, Osetek JD, Jones PB, Stern EA, Bacskai BJ, et al. Impaired spine stability underlies plaque-related spine loss in an Alzheimer's disease mouse model. *The American journal of pathology*. 2007;171(4):1304-11. Epub 2007/08/25.

[39] Kawahara M, Kuroda Y. Molecular mechanism of neurodegeneration induced by Alzheimer's beta-amyloid protein: channel formation and disruption of calcium homeostasis. *Brain research bulletin*. 2000;53(4):389-97. Epub 2001/01/04.

[40] Valincius G, Heinrich F, Budvytyte R, Vanderah DJ, McGillivray DJ, Sokolov Y, et al. Soluble amyloid beta-oligomers affect dielectric membrane properties by bilayer insertion and domain formation: implications for cell toxicity. *Biophysical journal*. 2008;95(10):4845-61. Epub 2008/06/03.

[41] Renner M, Lacor PN, Velasco PT, Xu J, Contractor A, Klein WL, et al. Deleterious effects of amyloid beta oligomers acting as an extracellular scaffold for mGluR5. *Neuron*. 2010;66(5):739-54. Epub 2010/06/16.

[42] Kamenetz F, Tomita T, Hsieh H, Seabrook G, Borchelt D, Iwatsubo T, et al. APP processing and synaptic function. *Neuron*. 2003;37(6):925-37. Epub 2003/04/03.

[43] Wei W, Nguyen LN, Kessels HW, Hagiwara H, Sisodia S, Malinow R. Amyloid beta from axons and dendrites reduces local spine number and plasticity. *Nature neuroscience*. 2010;13(2):190-6. Epub 2009/12/29.

[44] Hsieh H, Boehm J, Sato C, Iwatsubo T, Tomita T, Sisodia S, et al. AMPAR removal underlies Abeta-induced synaptic depression and dendritic spine loss. *Neuron*. 2006;52(5):831-43. Epub 2006/12/06.

[45] Nimmrich V, Grimm C, Draguhn A, Barghorn S, Lehmann A, Schoemaker H, et al. Amyloid beta oligomers (A beta(1-42) globulomer) suppress spontaneous synaptic activity by inhibition of P/Q-type calcium currents. *The Journal of neuroscience : the official journal of the Society for Neuroscience*. 2008;28(4):788-97. Epub 2008/01/25.

[46] Dixit R, Ross JL, Goldman YE, Holzbaur EL. Differential regulation of dynein and kinesin motor proteins by tau. *Science*. 2008; 319(5866):1086-9. Epub 2008/01/19.

[47] Mandelkow EM, Stamer K, Vogel R, Thies E, Mandelkow E. Clogging of axons by tau, inhibition of axonal traffic and starvation of synapses. *Neurobiology of aging*. 2003;24(8):1079-85. Epub 2003/12/04.

[48] Fulga TA, Elson-Schwab I, Khurana V, Steinhilb ML, Spires TL, Hyman BT, et al. Abnormal bundling and accumulation of F-actin mediates tau-induced neuronal degeneration in vivo. *Nature cell biology*. 2007;9(2):139-48. Epub 2006/12/26.

[49] Yoshiyama Y, Higuchi M, Zhang B, Huang SM, Iwata N, Saido TC, et al. Synapse loss and microglial activation precede tangles in a P301S tauopathy mouse model. *Neuron*. 2007;53(3):337-51. Epub 2007/02/03.

[50] Hoover BR, Reed MN, Su J, Penrod RD, Kotilinek LA, Grant MK, et al. Tau mislocalization to dendritic spines mediates synaptic dysfunction independently of neurodegeneration. *Neuron*. 2010;68(6):1067-81. Epub 2010/12/22.

[51] Chin J, Palop JJ, Puolivali J, Massaro C, Bien-Ly N, Gerstein H, et al. Fyn kinase induces synaptic and cognitive impairments in a transgenic mouse model of Alzheimer's disease. *The Journal of neuroscience : the official journal of the Society for Neuroscience*. 2005;25(42):9694-703. Epub 2005/10/21.

[52] Tu W, Xu X, Peng L, Zhong X, Zhang W, Soundarapandian MM, et al. DAPK1 interaction with NMDA receptor NR2B subunits mediates brain damage in stroke. *Cell*. 2010;140(2):222-34. Epub 2010/02/10.

[53] Liu Y, Wong TP, Aarts M, Rooyakkers A, Liu L, Lai TW, et al. NMDA receptor subunits have differential roles in mediating excitotoxic neuronal death both in vitro and in vivo. *The Journal of neuroscience :*

the official journal of the Society for Neuroscience. 2007;27(11):2846-57. Epub 2007/03/16.

[54] Yoneda S, Hara H, Hirata A, Fukushima M, Inomata Y, Tanihara H. Vitreous fluid levels of beta-amyloid((1-42)) and tau in patients with retinal diseases. *Japanese journal of ophthalmology*. 2005;49(2):106-8. Epub 2005/04/20.

[55] McKinnon SJ. Glaucoma: ocular Alzheimer's disease? *Frontiers in bioscience : a journal and virtual library*. 2003;8:s1140-56. Epub 2003/09/06.

[56] Kipfer-Kauer A, McKinnon SJ, Frueh BE, Goldblum D. Distribution of amyloid precursor protein and amyloid-beta in ocular hypertensive C57BL/6 mouse eyes. *Current eye research*. 2010;35(9):828-34. Epub 2010/08/28.

[57] Guo L, Salt TE, Luong V, Wood N, Cheung W, Maass A, et al. Targeting amyloid-beta in glaucoma treatment. *Proceedings of the National Academy of Sciences of the United States of America*. 2007;104(33):13444-9. Epub 2007/08/09.

[58] Gupta N, Fong J, Ang LC, Yucel YH. Retinal tau pathology in human glaucomas. Canadian journal of ophthalmology *Journal canadien d'ophtalmologie*. 2008;43(1):53-60. Epub 2008/01/26.

[59] Shankar GM, Bloodgood BL, Townsend M, Walsh DM, Selkoe DJ, Sabatini BL. Natural oligomers of the Alzheimer amyloid-beta protein induce reversible synapse loss by modulating an NMDA-type glutamate receptor-dependent signaling pathway. *The Journal of neuroscience : the official journal of the Society for Neuroscience*. 2007;27(11):2866-75. Epub 2007/03/16.

[60] Fu QL, Li X, Shi J, Xu G, Wen W, Lee DH, et al. Synaptic degeneration of retinal ganglion cells in a rat ocular hypertension glaucoma model. *Cellular and molecular neurobiology*. 2009;29(4):575-81. Epub 2009/01/28.

[61] Georgiou AL, Guo L, Cordeiro MF, Salt TE. Changes in NMDA receptor contribution to synaptic transmission in the brain in a rat model of glaucoma. *Neurobiology of disease*. 2010;39(3):344-51. Epub 2010/05/11.

[62] Crish SD, Sappington RM, Inman DM, Horner PJ, Calkins DJ. Distal axonopathy with structural persistence in glaucomatous neurodegeneration. *Proceedings of the National Academy of Sciences of the United States of America*. 2010;107(11):5196-201. Epub 2010/03/03.

[63] Ahmed F, Brown KM, Stephan DA, Morrison JC, Johnson EC, Tomarev SI. Microarray analysis of changes in mRNA levels in the rat retina after experimental elevation of intraocular pressure. *Investigative ophthalmology and visual science*. 2004;45(4):1247-58. Epub 2004/03/24.

[64] Kim HS, Park CK. Retinal ganglion cell death is delayed by activation of retinal intrinsic cell survival program. *Brain research*. 2005;1057(1-2):17-28. Epub 2005/09/06.

[65] Kuehn MH, Kim CY, Ostojic J, Bellin M, Alward WL, Stone EM, et al. Retinal synthesis and deposition of complement components induced by ocular hypertension. *Experimental eye research*. 2006;83(3):620-8. Epub 2006/05/09.

[66] Stasi K, Nagel D, Yang X, Wang RF, Ren L, Podos SM, et al. Complement component 1Q (C1Q) upregulation in retina of murine, primate, and human glaucomatous eyes. *Investigative ophthalmology and visual science*. 2006;47(3):1024-9. Epub 2006/03/01.

[67] Steele MR, Inman DM, Calkins DJ, Horner PJ, Vetter ML. Microarray analysis of retinal gene expression in the DBA/2J model of glaucoma. *Investigative ophthalmology and visual science*. 2006;47(3):977-85. Epub 2006/03/01.

[68] Stevens B, Allen NJ, Vazquez LE, Howell GR, Christopherson KS, Nouri N, et al. The classical complement cascade mediates CNS synapse elimination. *Cell*. 2007;131(6):1164-78. Epub 2007/12/18.

[69] Weber AJ, Chen H, Hubbard WC, Kaufman PL. Experimental glaucoma and cell size, density, and number in the primate lateral geniculate nucleus. *Investigative ophthalmology and visual science*. 2000;41(6):1370-9. Epub 2000/05/08.

[70] Weber AJ, Harman CD. Structure-function relations of parasol cells in the normal and glaucomatous primate retina. *Investigative ophthalmology and visual scien*ce. 2005;46(9):3197-207. Epub 2005/08/27.

[71] Shou T, Liu J, Wang W, Zhou Y, Zhao K. Differential dendritic shrinkage of alpha and beta retinal ganglion cells in cats with chronic glaucoma. *Investigative ophthalmology and visual science*. 2003;44(7):3005-10. Epub 2003/06/26.

[72] Morgan JE, Uchida H, Caprioli J. Retinal ganglion cell death in experimental glaucoma. *The British journal of ophthalmology*. 2000;84(3):303-10. Epub 2000/02/24.

[73] Gupta N, Ly T, Zhang Q, Kaufman PL, Weinreb RN, Yucel YH. Chronic ocular hypertension induces dendrite pathology in the lateral geniculate nucleus of the brain. *Experimental eye research.* 2007;84(1):176-84. Epub 2006/11/11.

[74] Watts RJ, Hoopfer ED, Luo L. Axon pruning during Drosophila metamorphosis: evidence for local degeneration and requirement of the ubiquitin-proteasome system. *Neuron.* 2003;38(6):871-85. Epub 2003/06/24.

[75] Kuo CT, Zhu S, Younger S, Jan LY, Jan YN. Identification of E2/E3 ubiquitinating enzymes and caspase activity regulating Drosophila sensory neuron dendrite pruning. *Neuron.* 2006;51(3):283-90. Epub 2006/08/02.

[76] Wagner MC, Pfister KK, Bloom GS, Brady ST. Copurification of kinesin polypeptides with microtubule-stimulated Mg-ATPase activity and kinetic analysis of enzymatic properties. *Cell motility and the cytoskeleton.* 1989;12(4):195-215. Epub 1989/01/01.

[77] Elluru RG, Bloom GS, Brady ST. Fast axonal transport of kinesin in the rat visual system: functionality of kinesin heavy chain isoforms. *Molecular biology of the cell.* 1995;6(1):21-40. Epub 1995/01/01.

[78] Masliah E, Hansen L, Albright T, Mallory M, Terry RD. Immunoelectron microscopic study of synaptic pathology in Alzheimer's disease. *Acta neuropathologica.* 1991;81(4):428-33. Epub 1991/01/01.

[79] Dessi F, Colle MA, Hauw JJ, Duyckaerts C. Accumulation of SNAP-25 immunoreactive material in axons of Alzheimer's disease. *Neuroreport.* 1997;8(17):3685-9. Epub 1998/01/14.

[80] Praprotnik D, Smith MA, Richey PL, Vinters HV, Perry G. Filament heterogeneity within the dystrophic neurites of senile plaques suggests blockage of fast axonal transport in Alzheimer's disease. *Acta neuropathologica.* 1996;91(3):226-35. Epub 1996/01/01.

[81] Pease ME, McKinnon SJ, Quigley HA, Kerrigan-Baumrind LA, Zack DJ. Obstructed axonal transport of BDNF and its receptor TrkB in experimental glaucoma. *Investigative ophthalmology and visual science.* 2000;41(3):764-74. Epub 2000/03/11.

[82] Coleman M. Molecular signaling how do axons die? *Advances in genetics.* 2011;73:185-217. Epub 2011/02/12.

[83] Hall AM, Roberson ED. Mouse models of Alzheimer's disease. *Brain research bulletin.* 2012;88(1):3-12. Epub 2011/12/07.

[84] Kanaan NM, Pigino GF, Brady ST, Lazarov O, Binder LI, Morfini GA. Axonal degeneration in Alzheimer's disease: When signaling

abnormalities meet the axonal transport system. *Experimental neurology*. 2012. Epub 2012/06/23.

[85] Pigino G, Morfini G, Atagi Y, Deshpande A, Yu C, Jungbauer L, et al. Disruption of fast axonal transport is a pathogenic mechanism for intraneuronal amyloid beta. *Proceedings of the National Academy of Sciences of the United States of America*. 2009;106(14):5907-12. Epub 2009/03/27.

[86] Decker H, Lo KY, Unger SM, Ferreira ST, Silverman MA. Amyloid-beta peptide oligomers disrupt axonal transport through an NMDA receptor-dependent mechanism that is mediated by glycogen synthase kinase 3beta in primary cultured hippocampal neurons. *The Journal of neuroscience : the official journal of the Society for Neuroscience*. 2010;30(27):9166-71. Epub 2010/07/09.

[87] Rui Y, Tiwari P, Xie Z, Zheng JQ. Acute impairment of mitochondrial trafficking by beta-amyloid peptides in hippocampal neurons. *The Journal of neuroscience : the official journal of the Society for Neuroscience*. 2006;26(41):10480-7. Epub 2006/10/13.

[88] LaPointe NE, Morfini G, Pigino G, Gaisina IN, Kozikowski AP, Binder LI, et al. The amino terminus of tau inhibits kinesin-dependent axonal transport: implications for filament toxicity. *Journal of neuroscience research*. 2009;87(2):440-51. Epub 2008/09/18.

[89] Sperber BR, Leight S, Goedert M, Lee VM. Glycogen synthase kinase-3 beta phosphorylates tau protein at multiple sites in intact cells. *Neuroscience letters*. 1995;197(2):149-53. Epub 1995/09/08.

[90] Kanaan NM, Morfini G, Pigino G, LaPointe NE, Andreadis A, Song Y, et al. Phosphorylation in the amino terminus of tau prevents inhibition of anterograde axonal transport. *Neurobiology of aging*. 2012;33(4):826 e15-30. Epub 2011/07/29.

[91] Takashima A, Murayama M, Murayama O, Kohno T, Honda T, Yasutake K, et al. Presenilin 1 associates with glycogen synthase kinase-3beta and its substrate tau. *Proceedings of the National Academy of Sciences of the United States of America*. 1998;95(16):9637-41. Epub 1998/08/05.

[92] Pigino G, Morfini G, Pelsman A, Mattson MP, Brady ST, Busciglio J. Alzheimer's presenilin 1 mutations impair kinesin-based axonal transport. *The Journal of neuroscience : the official journal of the Society for Neuroscience*. 2003;23(11):4499-508. Epub 2003/06/14.

[93] Song MS, Saavedra L, de Chaves EI. Apoptosis is secondary to non-apoptotic axonal degeneration in neurons exposed to Abeta in distal axons. *Neurobiology of aging*. 2006;27(9):1224-38. Epub 2005/08/27.
[94] Vosler PS, Brennan CS, Chen J. Calpain-mediated signaling mechanisms in neuronal injury and neurodegeneration. *Molecular neurobiology*. 2008;38(1):78-100. Epub 2008/08/08.
[95] Morgan JE, Jeffery G, Foss AJ. Axon deviation in the human lamina cribrosa. *The British journal of ophthalmology*. 1998;82(6):680-3. Epub 1998/11/03.
[96] Howell GR, Libby RT, Jakobs TC, Smith RS, Phalan FC, Barter JW, et al. Axons of retinal ganglion cells are insulted in the optic nerve early in DBA/2J glaucoma. *The Journal of cell biology*. 2007;179(7):1523-37. Epub 2007/12/26.
[97] Osborne NN, Melena J, Chidlow G, Wood JP. A hypothesis to explain ganglion cell death caused by vascular insults at the optic nerve head: possible implication for the treatment of glaucoma. *The British journal of ophthalmology*. 2001;85(10):1252-9. Epub 2001/09/25.
[98] Hernandez MR, Miao H, Lukas T. Astrocytes in glaucomatous optic neuropathy. *Progress in brain research*. 2008;173:353-73. Epub 2008/10/22.
[99] Libby RT, Li Y, Savinova OV, Barter J, Smith RS, Nickells RW, et al. Susceptibility to neurodegeneration in a glaucoma is modified by Bax gene dosage. *PLoS genetics*. 2005;1(1):17-26. Epub 2005/08/17.
[100] Knoferle J, Koch JC, Ostendorf T, Michel U, Planchamp V, Vutova P, et al. Mechanisms of acute axonal degeneration in the optic nerve in vivo. *Proceedings of the National Academy of Sciences of the United States of America*. 2010;107(13):6064-9. Epub 2010/03/17.
[101] Koch JC, Knoferle J, Tonges L, Ostendorf T, Bahr M, Lingor P. Acute axonal degeneration in vivo is attenuated by inhibition of autophagy in a calcium-dependent manner. *Autophagy*. 2010;6(5):658-9. Epub 2010/05/12.
[102] Tao J, Rolls MM. Dendrites have a rapid program of injury-induced degeneration that is molecularly distinct from developmental pruning. *The Journal of neuroscience : the official journal of the Society for Neuroscience*. 2011;31(14):5398-405. Epub 2011/04/08.
[103] Abramov AY, Scorziello A, Duchen MR. Three distinct mechanisms generate oxygen free radicals in neurons and contribute to cell death during anoxia and reoxygenation. *The Journal of neuroscience : the*

official journal of the Society for Neuroscience. 2007;27(5):1129-38. Epub 2007/02/03.

[104] Ward MW, Rego AC, Frenguelli BG, Nicholls DG. Mitochondrial membrane potential and glutamate excitotoxicity in cultured cerebellar granule cells. *The Journal of neuroscience : the official journal of the Society for Neuroscience*. 2000;20(19):7208-19. Epub 2000/09/29.

[105] Feng W, Liu G, Allen PD, Pessah IN. Transmembrane redox sensor of ryanodine receptor complex. *The Journal of biological chemistry*. 2000;275(46):35902-7. Epub 2000/09/22.

[106] Stasi K, Nagel D, Yang X, Ren L, Mittag T, Danias J. Ceruloplasmin upregulation in retina of murine and human glaucomatous eyes. *Investigative ophthalmology and visual science*. 2007;48(2):727-32. Epub 2007/01/26.

[107] Ghanem AA, Arafa LF, El-Baz A. Oxidative stress markers in patients with primary open-angle glaucoma. *Current eye research*. 2010;35(4):295-301. Epub 2010/04/09.

[108] Staal JA, Dickson TC, Gasperini R, Liu Y, Foa L, Vickers JC. Initial calcium release from intracellular stores followed by calcium dysregulation is linked to secondary axotomy following transient axonal stretch injury. *Journal of neurochemistry*. 2010;112(5):1147-55. Epub 2009/12/09.

[109] Sappington RM, Sidorova T, Long DJ, Calkins DJ. TRPV1: contribution to retinal ganglion cell apoptosis and increased intracellular Ca2+ with exposure to hydrostatic pressure. *Investigative ophthalmology and visual science*. 2009;50(2):717-28. Epub 2008/10/28.

[110] Buckingham BP, Inman DM, Lambert W, Oglesby E, Calkins DJ, Steele MR, et al. Progressive ganglion cell degeneration precedes neuronal loss in a mouse model of glaucoma. *The Journal of neuroscience : the official journal of the Society for Neuroscience*. 2008;28(11):2735-44. Epub 2008/03/14.

In: Recent Advances in Ophthalmology Research ISBN: 978-1-62808-021-6
Editor: Galina Dimitrova

Chapter 4

The Role of Innate Immunity in Dry Eye Syndrome

Laura Rania*[1*]*, Elisa Imelde Postorino*[1]*,
***Domenico Puzzolo*[2] *and Pasquale Aragona*[1]**
[1]Department of Surgical Specialties, Section of Ophthalmology, Ocular Surface Unit, University of Messina, Messina, Italy
[2]Department of Biomorphology and Biotechnologies, Section of Histology and Embryology, University of Messina, Messina, Italy

Abstract

Dry eye syndrome, (DE), also known as dysfunctional tear syndrome (DTS), is an inflammatory condition of the ocular surface derived by tear hyperosmolarity consequent to either increased tear evaporation (EDE) or aqueous deficiency (ADDE). Several external stimuli continuously trigger the ocular surface leading to a possible subclinical tissues inflammation, so that flogosis can be considered as a protective reaction against various noxae.

Both innate and adaptive immunity participate to the defensive systems of the ocular surface. Several mechanisms were indicated as promoters for innate immunity. Among these were described the altered

[*] Corresponding Author address: Department of Surgical Specialties, Section of Ophthalmology, University of Messina, Policlinico Universitario, I-98125, Messina, Italy. Email: ranialaura@libero.it.

production of various molecules (such as lactoferrin, lysozyme, lipocalin, secretory immunoglobulin A, acidic mammalian chitinase, phospholipase A2, transglutaminase 2) and the activation of toll-like receptors. Irritating stimuli, such as hyperosmolar tears, determine the interaction between the epithelial cells and receptors; this contact activate response pathways, such as mitogen-activated protein kinases, leading to the production of pro-inflammatory molecules. These events, occurring on both epithelial and dendritic cells, are responsible for the onset and maintaining of inflammation on the ocular surface.

Since an overlap of the two forms of DE is often present, it is difficult to differentiate between them. The finding of biomarkers that could help this differentiation would be of great relevance for the clinical practice. However, the dynamic evolution of the disease and the peculiar organization of the ocular surface render the identification of a single biomarker of the disease highly unlikely. Much more promising is the effort to identify molecules able to indicate a specific stage of a disease and a possible marker of therapeutic response.

Keywords: Dry eye, inflammation, immunity, ocular surface, inflammatory markers

Introduction

According to the definition and classification developed by the Dry Eye WorkShop in 2007, dry eye syndrome, (DE), also known as dysfunctional tear syndrome (DTS), is an inflammatory condition of the ocular surface derived by tear hyperosmolarity consequent to either increased tear evaporation (EDE) or aqueous deficiency (ADDE).

The Ocular Surface is a functional unit constituted by the epithelia of cornea, conjunctiva and lacrimal glands, lids (including the meibomian glands, the palpebral muscles, responsible for the blink, and the eyelashes with their associated glands of Moll and Zeis), sensory and motor nerves.

This functional unit is intended to protect the eye from the external environment and provide for an optimal refractive surface of the cornea through the production of an efficient tear film (Gipson 2007). The malfunctioning of one or more structures of the ocular surface determines compensatory changes of the others, in order to maintain an efficient tear film production. When a chronic alteration develops, the production of an efficient tear film will be impaired, configuring a dysfunctional tear syndrome.

Several external stimuli continuously trigger the ocular surface leading to a possible basal, subclinical response of the tissues towards inflammation, so that flogosis can be considered as a protective reaction against several stimuli.

Both innate and adaptive immunity participate to the defensive systems of the ocular surface. The innate mechanisms include the aberrant activation of toll-like receptors (TLRs), due to the modified ocular surface flora, and the increased expression of molecules, such as chitinases (AMCase), phospholipase A2 (PLA2) and transglutaminase 2 (TG2). These molecules were suggested as possible biomarkers for several inflammatory diseases.

The initiation of innate immunity mechanisms through these molecules results in the activation of the mitogen-activated protein kinase (MAPK) and nuclear factor kB (NF-kB) signaling pathways. This activation will induce the expression of pro-inflammatory cytokines such as interleukin (IL)-1α, IL-1β, tumor necrosis factor (TNF)-α and matrix metalloproteinases (MMP) (Li et al. 2004, Luo et al. 2005, De Paiva et al. 2006). The expression of these and other molecules triggers the consequent activation of the adaptive immune pathways and the maintenance of the inflammation onto the ocular surface. Whatever the initial cause of DE, the chronic irritation caused by the dysfunctional tear film results in excessive nervous stimulation aimed to induce compensatory responses, in order to achieve a functional recovery. The chronic nervous stimulation is responsible for neurogenic inflammation and T-cells activation with the release of inflammatory cytokines into the lacrimal glands, tears fluid and ocular surface epithelium. The ocular surface epithelial cells directly participate to the onset and maintenance of the inflammatory process by expressing on their membrane the antigens of Major Histocompatibility Complex-class II, such as HLA-DR (Tsubota et al. 1999, De Saint Jean et al. 1999), so acquiring antigen-presenting capability. In this way, epithelial cells either participate in the recruitment of inflammatory cells (dendritic cells, macrophages and lymphocytes) or become a target for cytotoxic reactions. These activities will result in epithelial suffering of lacrimal glands, cornea and conjunctiva. Another consequence of chronic inflammation of the ocular surface is the delivery, in the tear film, of pro-inflammatory molecules. These will stimulate a further expression of HLA-DR on cellular membranes and induce the epithelial cells apoptosis. This epithelial suffering is responsible for an altered mucin production, another cause of dysfunctional tear film.

The inflammatory mediators, deriving from the activity of infiltrating inflammatory cells, may determine a dysfunction of the ocular surface innervation. Consequently, a deprivation of the trophic signals for the lacrimal glands will result in lacrimal gland impairment and epithelial damage, due to the reduced delivery of trophic molecules, such as Epithelial Growth Factor (EGF), by the lacrimal gland itself. Once DE has developed, inflammation becomes the key mechanism of ocular surface injury, being both the origin and the result of cell damage. Therefore, patients with severe DE enter in a vicious cycle of inflammation and ocular surface injury (Wakamatsu et al. 2008).

The Molecular Basis of Innate Immunity

Several mechanisms were indicated as promoters for innate immunity. Among these were described the altered production of molecules such as lactoferrin, lysozyme, lipocalin (TLC), secretory immunoglobulin A (sIgA*)*, AMCase, PLA2, TG and the activation of TLRs.

Lactoferrin

Lactoferrin is an iron-binding, globular glycoprotein widely represented in tears. It has several functions, including anti-inflammatory effects, antibacterial, antiviral and anti-allergic functions. Lactoferrin can directly inhibit the production of several cytokines, such as TNF-α and IL-1. The antibacterial activity derives from deprivation of the bacterial flora from iron, an element necessary for its growth. Lactoferrin, mainly secreted from acinar cells of the lacrimal gland, is the main glycoprotein of tears. It possesses multiple functions including important bacteriostatic activity (Versura et al. 2010) and scavenging of free ions (Ohashi et al. 2003). Tear lactoferrin concentration has been shown to be a predictor of tear film stability or volume (Glasson et al. 2003), so that it represents an indicator of lacrimal secretory function. In fact, it has been considered a tear-specific biomarker for Sjögren's syndrome (SS). Furthermore, DE patients show a decreased concentration of lactoferrin in tears (Kawashima et al. 2012; Karns and Herr, 2011).

The level of tear lactoferrin can be correlated with the severity of corneo-conjunctival epithelial lesions in patients with primary and secondary SS, and non–SS DE. Since lactoferrin is largely related to the lacrimal tear function rather than Meibomian Gland Dysfunction (MGD), it was hypothesised that it may contribute to DE pathology via a non-MGD mechanism (Tong et al. 2011).

Lysozyme

Lysozyme is a glycoside hydrolase that damages bacterial cell walls by attacking their peptidoglycans. It is part of the innate immune system and is abundant in tears. Lysozyme, as well as lactoferrin, is produced in the acini of the main lacrimal gland, thus representing an indirect index of its function (Versura et al. 2010). The concentration of lysozyme decreases constantly in DE conditions. Moreover, it can vary according to age and different moments in a day. Lysozyme works sinergically with lactoferrin and tear lipocalin to enhance their efficacy. In fact, the activity of lysozyme could be inhibited by fatty acids secreted by the Meibomian glands and by nucleic acids. However, tear lipocalin can bind the long chain fatty acids, while lactoferrin binds nucleic acids. These bindings could result in an enhancement of lysozyme activity. In addition, tear lipocalin, lysozyme and lactoferrin could directly interact with each other (Dartt, 2011).

Lipocalins

The lipocalins are a broad family of various, low molecular weight proteins, which transport small hydrophobic molecules such as steroids, retinoids and lipids, including vitamin E and A. TLC can also bind to macromolecules, including the tear proteins lactoferrin and lysozyme (Dartt 2011). TLC is a multi-functional protein mainly secreted from the lacrimal gland into tear fluid, in addition with lysozyme and lactoferrin. TLC is the predominant lipid carrier in human tears and is second only to lysozyme, as the most concentrated protein. Lipocalins have been associated with many biological processes, such as the immune response, prostaglandin synthesis and retinoid binding.

TLC may regulate the lipid composition of tears by binding lipids from the tear fluid and/or releasing lipids into the tear fluid (Yamada et al. 2005). In fact, it scavenges lipids from the cornea, the conjunctiva and the tear film, as lipids render the corneal surface unwettable. On the other hand, it is able to deliver lipids, which participate to the non-Newtonian behaviour of tears (Dartt 2011). Lipocalins may also provide for a natural defence against fungal infections by binding to the microbial siderophores (iron scavenging molecules) (Glasgow and Gasymov 2011) and are the principal endonuclease in tears, being responsible for viral DNA inactivation (Dartt 2011).

TLC has been indicated as a biomarker of DE. In fact, it was demonstrated that its concentration is diminished or absent when lacrimal gland mass is reduced, or in disorders with an impaired lacrimal secretion, such as SS and LASIK induced DE (Glasgow and Gasymov 2011).

Immunoglobulin A (IgA)

Immunoglobulin A (IgA) is an antibody that plays a critical role in mucosal immunity. IgA can exist in a dimeric form called secretory IgA (sIgA). This represents the main immunoglobulin found in mucous secretions, including tears and saliva, and is produced by epithelial cells. It was demonstrated that in the condition of closed eyes secretory IgA represents the main tear protein, while lysozyme is the major protein in tears when eyes are opened. This is probably due to reflex tear production (Labbè et al. 2007). It was hypothesised that IgA could play a pivotal role in the pathogenesis of SS by representing a link between activated B cells and defective T cells. The high proportion of IgA in immunoglobulin production at the mucosal level supports this interpretation. It was reported that high levels of serum and secretory IgA, IgA-rheumatoid factor and IgA- containing circulating immune complexes are present in SS DE. A correlation between disease activity and the latter abnormalities has also been shown (Levy et al. 1994).

Acidic Mammalian Chitinase

Chitinases are endo-β-1,4 linked β-N-Acetyl-glucosaminidases. Recently, two distinct chitinases have been identified in humans: chitotriosidase (Chit), expressed in phagocytes, and an acidic mammalian chitinase (AMCase). The latter is expressed in allergic diseases of the gastrointestinal tract, lung and conjunctiva, as well as in the conjunctiva and tears of DE patients (Musumeci et al 2008). The levels of enzyme expression and the AMCase activity, in DE subjects, were different in MGD compared to SS patients (Musumeci et al. 2009). An explanation for this can be found in the different pathogenetic mechanism of the two forms. In MGD the altered tear film is characterized by a primary alteration of the lipid component, which can be accompanied by a modified bacterial flora on the conjunctiva (Dougherty and McCulley 1984). This might induce a stronger innate response as demonstrated by the higher AMCase expression level.

Phospholipase A2

PLA2 is a superfamily of enzymes that hydrolyze glycerophospholipids to produce lysophospholipids and free fatty acids (FFAs) (Wei et al. 2011). These latter include arachidonic acid, which is the precursor of inflammatory mediators, such as PGE2, leukotrienes and eicosaniods (Rosensons and Gelb 2009). Secretory PLA2 (sPLA2) plays a relevant role in the ocular innate immune defence system against Gram-positive bacteria and it has been reported that the level of sPLA2-IIa in normal human tears is at least 10,000 times higher than that in normal human serum (Aho et al. 2002). Furthermore, a role of sPLA2-IIa as an inflammatory mediator on the compromised ocular surface was suggested.

Transglutaminase-2

TG-2 is a ubiquitous protein which belongs to a family of calcium-dependent intra- and extracellular cross-linking enzymes.

It is regulated by cellular stress and participates in the induction of cell death (Png et al. 2011).

TG-2 plays the main role to ensure that once apoptosis has been initiated it is completed without causing inflammation and evident tissue injury. TG-2 can promote apoptosis (Tong et al. 2006) by either direct mechanism in certain apoptotic cells, or indirectly by promoting activation of transforming growth factor (TGF)-β released by macrophages. TG2-dependent cross-linking of proteins and formation of protective proteinaceous shells prevents the leakage of dangerous cellular products from the apoptotic cells, while TG-2 in macrophages promotes the speed of phagocytosis and results in further formation of TGF-β. If necrosis occurs, TG-2 promotes tissue stability and the subsequent repair.

Signaling Pathways

Irritating stimuli, such as hyperosmolar tears, determine the interaction of the epithelial cells with receptors. This action will activate response pathways, such as MAPKs, leading to the production of pro-inflammatory molecules. These events, occurring on both epithelial and dendritic cells, are responsible for the onset and maintaining of inflammation on the ocular surface (Pan et al. 2011).

Toll-like Receptors

TLRs are type I transmembrane glycoproteins which have two domains: one extracellular, leucine-rich, the other cytoplasmic which is homologous to that of the IL-1 receptor, hence referred to as the Toll/IL-1 receptor (TIR) domain. This mediates the activation of intracellular signaling pathways leading to functional changes including cytokines, chemokines and adhesion molecules expression. TLRs are key regulators of both innate and adaptive immune responses. They are thought to play a role in DE pathogenesis as the consequence of the modified ocular surface flora (Graham et al. 2007, Pflugfelder and Stern 2009).

TLRs primarily activate the innate immune response and mediate neutrophil infiltration to the tissues; they participate in surveillance system to control infection and tissue injury. On the other hand, TLR activation by endogenous ligands is associated with the development of autoimmune disorders, such as human systemic lupus erythematosus (Lamphier et al. 2006).

MAPKs /NF-kB

MAPKs are a family of serine/threonine protein kinases that play a central role in integrating the signals from a diverse group of extracellular stimuli and proto-oncogenes to the nucleus, affecting cell proliferation, differentiation, movement and death. MAPKs signaling pathways are organized hierarchically into three-tiered modules. MAP kinases (MAPKs) are phosphorylated and activated by MAP kinase kinases (MAPKKs), which are phosphorylated and activated by MAP kinase kinase kinases (MAPKKKs). The MAPKKKs are activated by the interaction with a family of small GTPases or other protein kinases connecting the MAP kinase pathway to cell surface receptors and thus to the external stimuli (Extracellular signal-regulated kinases - ERK).

The family of MAPKs (Qi and Elion 2005) therefore includes:

- ERK1 and ERK2, the "classical" MAPKs, regulate proliferation and differentiation and are activated in response to growth factors and cytokines, which stimulate a variety of receptors and G proteins.
- c-Jun N-terminal kinases (JNKs), (MAPK8, MAPK9, MAPK10), also known as stress- activated protein kinases (SAPKs), play crucial roles in regulating responses to various stresses, in inflammation and apoptosis.

p38 isoforms [p38-α (MAPK14), -β (MAPK11), -γ (MAPK12 or ERK6) and -δ (MAPK13 or SAPK4)] play an important role in human asthma and autoimmunity and are activated by numerous physical and chemical stresses, including hormones, UV irradiation, cytokines such as IL-1 and TNF, osmotic and heat shock.

Other members of the MAPK family are ERK3 (MAPK6), ERK4 (MAPK4), ERK5 (MAPK7), and ERK7/8 (MAPK15), whose role in dry eye has not been demonstrated.

NF-kB is a pleiotropic transcription factor that plays a critical role in the regulation of the expression of multiple genes involved in inflammatory responses (Zerfaoui et al. 2008).

NF-kB is important in regulating cellular responses because it belongs to the category of "rapid-acting" primary transcription factors, that is transcription factors that are present in cells in an inactive state and do not require new protein synthesis to be activated. This allows NF-kB to be a first responder to harmful cellular stimuli.

Pro-inflammatory Proteins

Interleukin-1

IL-1 is a powerful pro-inflammatory cytokine, which can be produced by many cell types, including macrophages, monocytes, lymphocytes, keratinocytes and fibroblasts in response to inflammation, infection, injury or other environmental stimuli (Dinarello 2011). Two isoforms, α and β, and a specific receptor antagonist, IL-1RA, have been described. Furthermore, two receptors for IL-1, a signaling receptor named IL-1RI and a decoy receptor named IL-1RII have been demonstrated (Zoukhri et al. 2007). Activation of the IL-1RI triggers a signaling cascade leading to the transcription of several genes involved in acute and chronic inflammation.

IL-1 is a potent inducer of other inflammatory cytokines such as IL-6 and -8, TNF-α, and granulocyte-macrophage colony-stimulating factor (GM-CSF). It also stimulates the production of MMP enzymes by epithelial and inflammatory cells. IL-1 has been implicated in the pathogenesis of corneal and ocular surface diseases, such as rosacea, bullous keratopathy, keratoconus and sterile corneal ulceration. DE is accompanied by an increase in the pro-inflammatory forms of IL-1 (both IL-1α and mature IL-1β) and a decrease in the biologically inactive precursor IL-1β in tear fluid.

Increased protease activity on the ocular surface may be one mechanism by which the precursor IL-1 β is cleaved to the mature, biologically active form. The conjunctival epithelium appears to be one source of the increased concentration of IL-1 in the tear fluid of patients with DE, so that IL-1 may play a key role in the pathogenesis of keratoconjunctivitis sicca (KCS) (Solomon et al. 2001).

Interleukin-2

Interleukin-2 (IL-2) is a signaling molecule of the immune system that attracts lymphocytes through its receptors (IL-2R), expressed by lymphocytes themselves. The bound of antigens to the T cell receptor (TCR) stimulates the secretion of IL-2 and the expression of its receptors leading thus to the growth, differentiation and survival of antigen- selected cytotoxic T cells via the activation of the expression of specific genes.

IL-2 is necessary for the development of T cell immunologic memory and the maturation of T- regs. In addition, it is required to discriminate between self and non-self. It was shown that in the tears of dry eye patients the concentration of IL-2 was increased. This augmentation is the result of an overproduction, rather than of evaporative effects, as suggested by an up-regulation of its gene in the conjunctiva (Massingale et al. 2009).

Interleukin-6

IL-6 is important for B cell growth and differentiation. It has a role in T cell stimulation and recruitment, since it promotes the transition of naive T cells to cytotoxic T cells. It also up-regulates ICAM-1, which functions as a receptor for activated T cells and, on many cells, as a co-stimulatory molecule for B cells (Roescher et al. 2009).

It was reported an increase of IL-6 in the tears of patients with mild to moderate EDE, thus demonstrating that inflammation plays a role not only in severe DE, but also in moderate EDE (Enriquez-de-Salamanca et al. 2010)and recent reports include observations of increased IL-6 levels in patients with KCS, keratoconus, and conjunctivo-chalasis, such as in the tears of patients suffering from ADDE compared to healthy volunteers (Yoon et al. 2007).

Interleukin-17

Interleukin-17 (IL-17 or IL-17A), a potent pro-inflammatory cytokine produced by activated memory T cells, is the founding member of a group of cytokines called the IL-17 family (Gurney and Aggarwal 2002). It acts by increasing chemokine production in various tissues to recruit monocytes and neutrophils to the site of inflammation, similar to Interferon (IFN)-γ; furthermore it acts synergistically with TNF and IL-1 (Miossec et al. 2009). IL-17 works by binding to a type I cell surface receptor called IL-17R. IL-17 induces the production of many other cytokines (such as IL-6, G-CSF, GM-CSF, IL-1β, TGF-β, TNF-α), chemokines (including IL-8, CXCL1, and CCL2), MMPs and PGE2 from many cell types (fibroblasts, endothelial cells, epithelial cells and macrophages). The increased expression of chemokines attracts other cells, including neutrophils, but not eosinophils. IL-17 function is also essential to a subset of CD4+ T-Cells called T helper 17 (Th17) cells. As a result of these roles, the IL-17 family has been linked to many immune/autoimmune related diseases, including rheumatoid arthritis, allograft rejection and anti-tumour immunity (Kolls and Linden 2004).

The increased presence of IL-17 in the tears of DE patients (Chung et al. 2012), along with the demonstration of Th17 cells and expression of IL-17R by the ocular surface epithelia, indicates the importance of an IL-17-mediated cytokine cascade in the immunopathogenesis of DE. The constitutive expression of IL-17 receptors by corneal and conjunctival epithelia makes ocular surface more vulnerable to IL-17 mediated inflammation and tissue damage. The functional relevance of Th17 cells in the immunopathogenesis of DE is fundamentally confirmed by the finding that in vivo neutralization of IL-17 results in a markedly attenuated induction and severity of the disease (Kang et al. 2011).

Tumor Necrosis Factor-α

TNF-α is a cytokine involved in systemic inflammation and is a member of a group of cytokines that stimulate the acute phase reaction. TNF is produced primarily by macrophages, but also by a large variety of cell types, including lymphoid cells, mast cells, fibroblasts and epithelial cells. Large amounts of TNF are released in response to lipopolysaccharide, other bacterial products, and IL-1. The primary role of TNF is the regulation of immune cells activity.

TNF can bind two receptors, TNF-R1 (TNF receptor type 1; CD120a; p55/60) and TNF-R2 (TNF receptor type 2; CD120b; p75/80). In the ocular surface TNF-α is synthetized by mast cells, T lymphocytes and the majority of epithelial cells, so amplifying the role of these cells when involved in an inflammatory, toxic or degenerative process. TNF-α interacts with other cytokines, such as Fas ligand, IL1α and β or IFN-γ, thus leading to apoptosis and inflammation (Baudouin and Liang 2005) It has been implicated in the pathogenesis of corneal ulceration, uveitis, and corneal transplant rejection (Goyal et al. 2009). In fact, an increased production and activation of this cytokine has been demonstrated in various ocular surface diseases, including DE (Pflugfelder et al. 1999, VanDerMeid et al. 2011). In the latter condition the up-regulation of TNF-α gene in the conjunctiva suggests that the increased concentration in tears is not the result of evaporative effects, but of overproduction (Massingale et al. 2009). However, it has been shown that TNF- α level, unlike the one of IL-6, is not associated with the severity of the disease and does not correlate with various ocular surface parameters (Yoon et al. 2007). TNF-α has been found to affect neural sensitivity and to cause ocular surface hyperalgesia. In fact, it has been hypothesized that elevated tear cytokine concentrations, and TNF-α among these, might be a more sensitive disease marker, than traditional signs, in those patients with mild DE complaining of ocular discomfort despite the absence of objective signs (Lam et al. 2009).

Furthermore, differences were noted between the ADE and EDDE patients. In fact, in the latter group a lower TNF-α concentration was showed. This evidence led to the assumption that mechanisms other than inflammation can be responsible of dry eye in these patients (Boehm et al. 2011).

Interferon-γ

Interferon-gamma (IFN-γ), or type II interferon, is a dimerized soluble cytokine encoded by the IFNG gene. It plays a pivotal role in innate and adaptive immunity against viral and intracellular bacterial infections by direct inhibition of viral replication (Schoenborn and Wilson 2007). IFN-γ is secreted by T helper cells (Th1 cells), cytotoxic T cells (TC cells) and NK cells, while INF-α and INF-β can be expressed by every cell. IFN-γ produces a variety of physiological and cellular responses, such as the promotion of NK cell activity, the increase of antigen presentation and lysosomes activity in macrophages, the activation of inducible Nitric Oxide Synthase (iNOS) and the promotion of Th1 differentiation. Furthermore, it induces normal cells to increase expression of class I MHC molecules as well as class II MHC on antigen presenting cells. IFN-γ plays a crucial role in regulating several immune responses, such as delayed-type hypersensitivity, inflammation, graft rejection and the pathogenesis of inflammatory diseases (SS, mucus membrane pemphigoid, Stevens-Johnson syndrome, and graft-versus-host disease). In addition, it was demonstrated that desiccating stress promoted the migration of CD4+ T cells and IFN- γ expressing cells into the conjunctiva and increased the concentration of IFN- γ in tears in DE conditions. Increased IFN- γ can lead to conjunctival epithelial squamous metaplasia and to the pathologic apoptosis, characterized by increased Th- 1 and Th-17 CD4+ T cell infiltration on the ocular surface (Zhang et al. 2011).

Transforming Growth Factor –β

Transforming growth factor beta (TGF-β) is a pleiotropic cytokine that plays a crucial role in the regulation of the cell cycle. In fact, it directs cellular proliferation, differentiation, wound healing, inflammation and other functions in most cells. Furthermore, it induces apoptosis in numerous cell types. At least three isoforms of TGF-β are known, called TGF-β1, TGF-β2 and TGF-β3. TGF-β1 is the main member of this family. It regulates the expression of many other growth factors through the interaction with its receptors present on many cell types. Some cells that secrete TGF-β1 also have receptors for TGF-β1: this is known as autocrine signaling (Dogar et al. 2011).

Among the functions of TGF-β are: promoting the rate of apoptosis, through the induction of TG-2; increasing the efficiency of macrophages phagocytosis; down-regulating the production of pro-inflammatory cytokines in macrophages. TGF-β 1 is produced by the human lacrimal gland and corneal and conjunctival epithelia and has been detected in tears (Zheng et al. 2010). During corneal wound healing, TGF-β stimulates the synthesis of collagen, in addition to that of hyaluronan, biglycan, and fibronectin, components of the fibrotic extracellular matrix (Etheredge et al. 2010).

TGF- β activity is fundamental in the immune system of the ocular surface where it can play a dual role: first, it prevents the development of autoimmune reactions by blocking T and B cells proliferation and promoting the differentiation and activity of regulatory T cells (Tregs), so contributing to the homeostasis maintenance. On the other hand, TGF-β generates an immune response to stress, such as desiccation, which induces the generation of pathogenic IL-17-producing effector cells (Th-17) (De Paiva et al. 2011).

Matrix Metalloproteinases

Matrix metalloproteinases (MMPs) are a family of zinc- and calcium-dependent enzymes, involved in the breakdown of extracellular matrix in normal physiological processes, such as embryonic development, morphogenesis, reproduction, tissues resorption and remodeling. Moreover, they play an important role in various pathologic processes, such as inflammation, arthritis, cancer and different autoimmune diseases, including systemic lupus erythematosus, SS, systemic sclerosis and rheumatoid arthritis. MMP-9 is the most important gelatinase present on the ocular surface (Meloni et al. 2011) and its levels appear to be higher in tears of patients suffering from dry eye, the highest concentration being observed in SS, corneal epithelial defects and steril stromal ulcer. MMP-9 lyses a large number of substrates, including the components of the corneal epithelial basement membrane and the tight junction proteins (ZO-1 and occludin), thus compromising the integrity of the corneal epithelial barrier. MMP-9 appears to play a physiologic role in regulating corneal epithelial desquamation. Among its various activities, MMP-9 is known to activate precursor IL-1β and latent TGF-1β into their active forms. Therefore, the increase of MMP-9 activity on the ocular surface can amplify the chronic immune-based inflammation in DTS (Chotikavanich et al. 2009).

HLA-DR

HLA-DR is a α - β heterodimer, cell surface receptor, belonging to the MHC class II cell surface receptors encoded by the human leukocyte antigen complex.

The primary function of HLA-DR is to present peptide antigens, potentially foreign in origin, to the immune system in order to stimulate or suppress T-helper cell responses that eventually lead to the production of antibodies against the same antigens, so that it works as cell recruiting molecule. HLA-DR plays a critical role in the initiation of the immune response. An over-expression of HLA-DR has been demonstrated in the epithelial cells of both ocular and non-ocular tissues affected by inflammatory disorders (Versura et al. 2011); among the former are patients with SS, chronic conjunctivitis, and DE (Mrugacz and Zywalewska 2005). In particular, KCS and ocular rosacea were associated with over-expression of inflammatory markers such as HLA-DR and ICAM-1 and a significant decrease in the number of goblet cells (Pisella et al. 2001).

HLA-DR antigen measurement might be a useful method for monitoring inflammatory conjunctival changes in DE, as it has been showed that its increased expression positively correlates with the parameters of DE diagnostic tests.

Chemokines

Chemokines are low molecular weight proteins, secreted by cells, which play important roles in physiologic mechanisms and in the regulation of inflammatory responses (Barabino and Dana 2007). They serve to guide cells of both innate and adaptive immune system and are implicated in the ocular surface disorders occurring in DE.

Inflammatory chemokines are released from a wide variety of cells in response to bacterial or viral infections, or to agents that cause physical damage; their release is often stimulated by pro-inflammatory cytokines, such as IL-1. They function mainly as chemoattractants for leukocytes, recruiting monocytes, neutrophils and other cells from the blood to sites of infection or tissue damage, and put forth their biological effects by interacting with transmembrane receptors (chemokine receptors).

Adhesion Molecules (ICAM-1, VCAM-1)

Cellular adhesion molecules (CAMs) play a primary role in cell-cell recognition. They are cell surface proteins that facilitate cellular migration by binding to extracellular matrix components; in DE patients intercellular adhesion molecules (ICAMs) and vascular cell adhesion molecules (VCAMs) have been identified in the conjunctiva and the lacrimal gland.

ICAMs are cell surface glycoproteins expressed on leukocytes, epithelial cells, endothelial cells and fibroblasts. Five ICAMs have been identified, and ICAM-1 (CD54) is the most studied. Stimulation with inflammatory cytokines such as IL-1, TNF-α, and IFN-γ or with CD40 has been shown to increase ICAM-1 in many cell types.

VCAM-1 is a cell surface glycoprotein involved in the recruitment and binding of lymphocytes, monocytes, eosinophils, and basophils to the vascular endothelium. It is over-expressed in all DE disorders owing to the presence of lymphocyte activation. Pro-inflammatory neurotransmitters, such as substance P, lead to ICAM-1 and VCAM-1 expression, so promoting lymphocyte homing and chemotaxis to sites of inflammation.

Conclusion

Both forms of DE, ADDE and EDE, can be considered as models for inflammatory ocular surface disease. Since an overlap of the two forms is often present, it is difficult to differentiate between them. The finding of biomarkers that could help this differentiation would be of great relevance for the clinical practice. Moreover, diagnostic biomarkers should allow a differentiation between patients and normals, but also from other diseases with overlapping characteristics, for example seasonal allergic conjunctivitis (SAC). Several functions can be attributed to a biomarker: individuate people at risk to develop the disease; screen and diagnose a disease; scale its severity; monitor the progress or the remission phases; predict the response to the therapy; determine the prognosis and contribute to understand the disease pathophysiology. Any measurable, disease-associated, biological parameter could be a biomarker. It would be of interest to know about the risk to develop DE in predisposing circumstances, for example in course of both topical or systemic conditions such as: contact lens wear; refractive laser surgery; chronic use of preserved eye drops (e.g. in glaucoma treatment); postmenopausal oestrogen therapy; chronic use of systemic therapies like antihistamines, beta-blockers, diuretics; connective tissue diseases; graft versus host diseases after bone marrow transplantation; androgen deficiency or androgen receptor blockade. Biomarkers correlating with symptoms would be of interest, as well as molecules that, even if not correlating with symptoms, may characterize other features of the disease, such as inflammation, and may be a confirmation of intrinsic mechanisms. Although the pathophysiological mechanisms of ocular surface inflammation have been convincingly elucidated, there is a lack of biomarkers representing a specific pattern for each clinical type of DE. Under this aspect, biomarkers deriving from the inflammatory pathways may be useful to identify a specific stage of the disease, rather than be used as an indicator of a specific clinical subtype of DE. The dynamic evolution of ocular surface responses to the various noxae and the peculiar organization of the ocular surface functional unit render the identification of a single biomarker of the disease highly unlikely. Much more promising is the effort to identify molecules able to indicate a specific stage of a disease and a possible marker of therapeutic response.

References

Aho VV, Nevalainen TJ, Saari KM. Group IIA phospholipase A2 content of tears in patients with keratoconjunctivitis sicca. *Graefes Arch Clin Exp Ophthalmol* 2002;240:521-523.

Barabino S, Dana MR. Dry eye syndromes. *Chem Immunol Allergy* 2007;92:176-184.

Baudouin C, Liang H. Amplifying factors in ocular surface diseases: apoptosis. *Ocul Surf* 2005;3:S194-197.

Boehm N, Riechardt AI, Wiegand M, et al. Proinflammatory cytokine profiling of tears from dry eye patients by means of antibody microarrays. *Invest Ophthalmol Vis Sci* 2011;52:7725-7730.

Chotikavanich S, de Paiva CS, Li de Q, et al. Production and activity of matrix metalloproteinase-9 on the ocular surface increase in dysfunctional tear syndrome. *Invest Ophthalmol Vis Sci* 2009;50:3203-3209.

Chung JK, Kim MK, Wee WR. Prognostic factors for the clinical severity of keratoconjunctivitis sicca in patients with Sjögren's syndrome. *Br J Ophthalmol* 2012;96:240-245.

Dartt DA. Tear lipocalin: structure and function. *Ocul Surf* 2011;9:126-138.

De Paiva CS, Corrales RM, Villarreal AL, et al. Corticosteroid and doxycycline suppress MMP-9 and inflammatory cytokine expression,

MapK activation in the corneal epithelium in experimental dry eye. *Exp Eye Res* 2006;83:526-535.

De Paiva CS, Volpe EA, Gandhi NB, et al. Disruption of TGF-β signaling improves ocular surface epithelial disease in experimental autoimmune keratoconjunctivitis sicca. *PLoS One* 2011;6:e29017.

De Saint Jean M, Brignole F, Feldmann G, et al. Interferon-gamma induces apoptosis and expression of inflammation-related proteins in Chang conjunctival cells. *Invest Ophthalmol Vis Sci* 1999;40:2199-2212.

Dinarello CA. Interleukin-1 in the pathogenesis and treatment of inflammatory diseases *Blood* 2011;117:3720-3732.

Dogar AM, Towbin H, Hall J. Suppression of latent transforming growth factor (TGF)-beta1 restores growth inhibitory TGF-beta signaling through microRNAs. *J Biol Chem* 2011;286:16447-16458.

Dougherty JM, McCulley JP. Comparative bacteriology of chronic blepharitis. *Br J Ophthalmol* 1984;68:524-528.

Enriquez-de-Salamanca A, Castellanos E, Stern ME, et al. Tear cytokine and chemokine analysis and clinical correlations in evaporative-type dry eye disease. *Mol Vis* 2010;16:862-873.

Etheredge L, Kane BP, Valkov N, et al. Enhanced cell accumulation and collagen processing by keratocytes cultured under agarose and in media containing IGF-I, TGF-β or PDGF. *Matrix Biol* 2010;29:519-524.

Gipson IK. The ocular surface: the challenge to enable and protect vision: the Friedenwald lecture. *Invest Ophthalmol Vis Sci* 2007;48:4391-4398.

Glasgow BJ, Gasymov OK. Focus on molecules: tear lipocalin. *Exp Eye Res* 2011;92:242-243.

Glasson MJ, Stapleton F, Keay L, et al. Differences in clinical parameters and tear film of tolerant and intolerant contact lens wearers. *Invest Ophthalmol Vis Sci* 2003;44:5116-5124.

Goyal S, Chauhan SK, Zhang Q, Dana R. Amelioration of murine dry eye disease by topical antagonist to chemokine receptor 2. *Arch Ophthalmol* 2009;127:882-887.

Graham JE, Moore JE, Jiru X, et al. Ocular pathogen or commensal: a PCR-based study of surface bacterial flora in normal and dry eyes. *Invest Ophthalmol Vis Sci* 2007;48:5616-5623.

Gurney AL, Aggarwal S. IL-17: prototype member of an emerging cytokine family. *J Leukoc Biol* 2002;71:1-8.

Kang MH, Kim MK, Lee HJ, et al. Interleukin-17 in various ocular surface inflammatory diseases. *J Korean Med Sci* 2011;26:938-944.

Karns K, Herr AE. Human tear protein analysis enabled by an alkaline microfluidic homogeneous immunoassay. *Anal Chem* 2011;83:8115-8122.

Kawashima M, Kawakita T, Inaba T, et al. Dietary lactoferrin alleviates age-related lacrimal gland dysfunction in mice. *PLoS One* 2012;7:e33148.

Kolls JK, Linden A. Interleukin-17 family members and inflammation. *Immunity* 2004;21:467-476.

Labbé A, Brignole-Baudouin F, Baudouin C. Ocular surface investigations in dry eye. *J Fr Ophtalmol* 2007;30:76-97.

Lam H, Bleiden L, de Paiva CS, et al. Tear cytokine profiles in dysfunctional tear syndrome. *Am J Ophthalmol* 2009;147:198-205.

Lamphier MS, Sirois CM, Verma A, et al. TLR9 and the recognition of self and non-self nucleic acids. *Ann N Y Acad Sci* 2006;1082:31-43.

Levy Y, Dueymes M, Pennec YL, et al. IgA in Sjögren's syndrome. *Clin Exp Rheumatol* 1994;12:543-551.

Li DQ, Chen Z, Song XJ, et al. Stimulation of matrix metalloproteinases by hyperosmolarity via a JNK pathway in human corneal epithelial cells. *Invest Ophthalmol Vis Sci* 2004;45:4302-4311.

Luo L, Li DQ, Corrales RM, et al. Hyperosmolar saline is a proinflammatory stress on the mouse ocular surface. *Eye Contact Lens* 2005;31:186-193.

Massingale ML, Li X, Vallabhajosyula M, et al. Analysis of inflammatory cytokines in the tears of dry eye patients. *Cornea* 2009;28:1023-1027.

Meloni M, De Servi B, Marasco D, Del Prete S. Molecular mechanism of ocular surface damage: application to an in vitro dry eye model on human corneal epithelium. *Mol Vis* 2011;17:113-126.

Miossec P, Korn T, Kuchroo VK. Interleukin-17 and type 17 helper T cells. *N Engl J* Med 2009;361:888- 898.

Mrugacz M, Zywalewska N. HLA-DR antigen expression on conjunctival epithelial cells in patients with dry eye. *Klin Oczna* 2005;107:278-279.

Musumeci M, Bellin M, Maltese A et al. Chitinase levels in the tears of subjects with ocular allergies. *Cornea* 2008;27(2):168-73.

Musumeci M, Bellin M, Maltese A et al. Chitinase levels in the tears of subjects with ocular allergies. Cornea 2008;27(2):168-73.

Musumeci M, Aragona P, Bellin M, et al. Acidic mammalian chitinase in dry eye conditions. *Cornea* 2009;28:667-672.

Ohashi Y, Ishida R, Kojima T, et al. Abnormal protein profiles in tears with dry eye syndrome. *Am J Ophthalmol* 2003;136:291-299.

Pan Z, Wang Z, Yang H, et al. TRPV1 activation is required for hypertonicity-stimulated inflammatory cytokine release in human corneal epithelial cells. Invest Ophthalmol Vis Sci 2011;52:485-493.

Pflugfelder SC, Jones D, Ji Z, et al. Altered cytokine balance in the tear fluid and conjunctiva of patients with Sjögren's syndrome keratoconjunctivitis sicca. *Curr Eye Res* 1999;19:201-211.

Pflugfelder SC, Stern ME. Immunoregulation on the ocular surface: 2nd Cullen Symposium. *Ocul Surf* 2009;7:67-77.

Pisella PJ, Malet F, Lejeune S, et al. Ocular surface changes induced by contact lens wear. *Cornea* 2001;20:820-825.

Png E, Samivelu GK, Yeo SH, et al. Hyperosmolarity-mediated mitochondrial dysfunction requires Transglutaminase-2 in human corneal epithelial cells. *J Cell Physiol* 2011;226:693-699.

Roescher N, Tak PP, Illei GG. Cytokines in Sjögren's syndrome. *Oral Diseases* 2009;15:519-526.

Rosenson RS, Gelb MH. Secretory phospholipase A2: a multifaceted family of proatherogenic enzymes. *Curr Cardiol Rep* 2009;11:445-451.

Schoenborn JR, Wilson CB. Regulation of interferon-gamma during innate and adaptive immune responses. *Adv Immunol* 2007;96:41-101.

Solomon A, Dursun D, Liu Z, et al. Pro- and anti-inflammatory forms of interleukin-1 in the tear fluid and conjunctiva of patients with dry-eye disease. *Invest Ophthalmol Vis Sci* 2001;42:2283-2292.

Tong L, Chen Z, De Paiva CS, et al. Transglutaminase participates in UVB-induced cell death pathways in human corneal epithelial cells. *Invest Ophthalmol Vis Sci* 2006;47:4295-4301.

Tong L, Zhou L, Beuerman RW, et al. Association of tear proteins with Meibomian gland disease and dry eye symptoms. *Br J Ophthalmol* 2011;95:848-852.

Tsubota K, Fukagawa K, Fujihara T, et al. Regulation of human leukocyte antigen expression in human conjunctival epithelium. *Invest Ophthalmol Vis Sci* 1999;40:28-34.

VanDerMeid KR, Su SP, Krenzer KL, et al. A method to extract cytokines and matrix metalloproteinases from Schirmer strips and analyze using Luminex. *Mol Vis* 2011;17:1056-1063.

Versura P, Nanni P, Bavelloni A, et al. Tear proteomics in evaporative dry eye disease. *Eye* 2010;24:1396- 1402.

Versura P, Profazio V, Schiavi C, Campos EC. Hyperosmolar stress upregulates HLA-DR expression in human conjunctival epithelium in dry eye patients and in vitro models. *Invest Ophthalmol Vis Sci* 2011;52:5488-5496.

Wakamatsu TH, Dogru M, Tsubota K. Tearful relations: oxidative stress, inflammation and eye diseases. *Arq Bras Oftalmol* 2008;71:72-79.

Wei Y, Epstein SP, Fukuoka S, et al. sPLA2-IIa amplifies ocular surface inflammation in the expérimental dry eye (DE) BALB/c mouse model. *Invest Ophthalmol Vis Sci* 2011;52:4780-4788.

Yoon KC, Jeong IY, Park YG, Yang SY. Interleukin-6 and tumor necrosis factor alpha levels in tears of patients with dry eye syndrome. *Cornea* 2007;26:431-437.

Zerfaoui M, Suzuki Y, Naura AS, et al. Nuclear translocation of p65 NF-kappaB is sufficient for VCAM-1, but not ICAM-1, expression in TNF-stimulated smooth muscle cells: differential requirement for PARP-1 expression and interaction. *Cell Signal* 2008;20:186-194.

Zhang X, Chen W, De Paiva CS, et al. Interferon-g exacerbates dry eye-induced apoptosis in conjunctiva through dual apoptotic pathways. *Invest Ophthalmol Vis Sci* 2011;52:6279-6285.

Zheng X, De Paiva CS, Rao K, et al. Evaluation of the transforming growth factor-beta activity in normal and dry eye human tears by CCL-185 cell bioassay. *Cornea* 2010;29:1048-1054.

Zoukhri D, Macari E, Kublin CL. A single injection of interleukin-1 induces reversible aqueous-tear deficiency, lacrimal gland inflammation, and acinar and ductal cell proliferation. *Exp Eye Res* 2007;84:894- 904.

In: Recent Advances in Ophthalmology Research ISBN: 978-1-62808-021-6
Editor: Galina Dimitrova

Chapter 5

Ocular Stem Cells: An Overview

Kamesh Dhamodaran, Reshma Shetty, Murali Subramani and Debashish Das*
Stem Cell Research Laboratory, Narayana Nethralaya, Bangalore, India

Abstract

The last two decades have added a new facet in the field of therapy in health sciences with the emergence of stem cells and regenerative medicine. This branch of regenerative medicine and its allied research have been advancing exponentially. The potentials and characteristics of these cells categorize them under a different group away from other cell types of the body. Stem cells represent unspecialized cells harboring properties for proliferation and differentiation that enable them to become tissue or organ specific cells. Stem cells are regarded as the future of medicine and looked up as a panacea for diseases. Research studies are underway worldwide for utilizing stem cells to treat diseases such as diabetes, Alzheimer's, Parkinson's, muscular dystrophy, spinal cord injury, etc. The routine use of stem cells must be highly regulated to prevent any kind of abuse to the potential of these incredible cells.

Among all the branches of health sciences, ophthalmology became the first to get the benefits of stem cell treatment. The eye, being an

* Corresponding author: Stem Cell Research Laboratory, Narayana Nethralaya Foundation, Narayana Health City. 258/A Bommsandra Industrial Area. Hosur Road, Bangalore 560099. Karanataka, India. dasdebashish@yahoo.co.uk; drdebashish@narayananethralaya.com.

immune privileged organ, fulfills all the necessary criteria for stem cell treatment and research. The eye is easily accessible to treatment, follow-up, and investigation of final outcome. First clinical trial of embryonic stem cells was done recently in diseased eye for two patients suffering from Stargardt's macular dystrophy and age-related macular dystrophy. The most wide and successful use of adult stem cells in treatment concerns limbal epithelial cell transplantation for removing corneal scar or patients with limbal stem cell deficiency.

Based on their origin, stem cells are generally classified into embryonic and adult stem cells. This chapter deals mostly with adult stem cells, although we also address some of the recent advances of embryonic stem cells research in ophthalmology. Major causes of blindness worldwide include abnormal vasculature, with or without neuronal degeneration. The use of stem/progenitor cells for remedy or prevention of ocular disease progression holds a great promise. Stem cell therapies have already been successfully used for treating the anterior surface of the cornea. Diseases pertaining to the posterior region of the eye such as degenerative diseases (inherited retinal degeneration, macular degeneration) or vascular diseases (diabetic retinopathy, retinopathy of prematurity, etc.) are more challenging to treat with cell-based therapy. The clinical utility of stem cells may be realized by their transplantation to the damaged part, through paracrine signals released from healthy cells/tissues or by providing guidance cues to attract endogenous circulating progenitor/stem cells. Ophthalmology leads the branch of regenerative medicine wherein stem cells have been used for therapy.

In this chapter, we have addressed the different aspects of usage of stem cells in treating ocular diseases, including the ongoing research efforts and the future prospects.

Keywords: Stem cells, regenerative medicine, ocular stem cells, limbus, retina

Introduction

Stem cells are identified by their characteristic property of self-renewal (proliferation) and differentiation. These cells, based on their origin, have been classified into embryonic stem cells and adult stem cells. The stem cells harbor a huge potential for therapeutic use in various pathologies because of their characteristic pluripotency. Embryonic stem cells are pluripotent, whereas adult stem cells are multipotent. However, the present technological advances in science have broken the barriers and can induce pluripotency to adult stem cells as well as to somatic cells.

Embryonic stem cells are collected from the inner cell mass at the gastrulation stage of a fertilized egg and are cultured under appropriate conditions to maintain pluripotency. These, under certain predefined conditions, can be differentiated to various cell lineages. The field of science and research revolving around embryonic stem cells has been marked with several religious scandals and ethical controversies. Hence, the field of embryonic stem cell research, though having had a huge therapeutic potential, was outpaced by adult stem cells research. Adult stem cells are multipotent in nature and are present more or less in almost all tissues of our body. Most commonly, adult stem cells are isolated from peripheral blood, bone marrow, and cord blood. These are a kind of progenitor/stem cells that under certain conditions can replace damaged cells.

Recent advances in stem cell research have widened the prospects of using cell-based therapies to regenerate irreversibly damaged ocular tissues by disease or injury. Among all the other parts of the body, the eye is the most privileged organ for stem cell-based therapy. Stem cell based therapy is practiced widely for regenerating human corneal epithelial tissues. The eye holds several advantages to be the first organ of choice for stem cell treatment. It is an immune privileged organ, in which it is easier to make follow-up for the clinical readout of the outcome. On the other hand, different parts of the eye derive from different types of embryonic tissues. The neurosensory retina and the retinal pigment epithelium derive from neuroectoderm; the mesoderm differentiates into the corneoscleral and uveal tunics, whereas the lens derives from ectoderm.

Hence, the feasibility, efficacy, and success of cell-based regeneration depend on the potential of the cells to differentiate into complex tissues. Repairing a damaged or scarred corneal surface is much easier regarding the epithelial nature of the cells, whereas repairing a damaged retina is more cumbersome because regenerated neurons need to integrate into an existing architecture and generate neuronal activity. In most of such cases, complex protocols and inter-disciplinary approaches are hybridized for a successful outcome.

Anatomical, as well as physiological abnormalities of the optical pathway, phototransduction pathway, neuronal pathways, or visual cortex can lead to blindness. There are different modes of using stem cells for treating ocular pathologies: (a) cell replacement using healthy cells generated from stem cells, (b) through the paracrine effect wherein the niche is maintained healthy, (c) providing guidance cues to attract circulating progenitor cells to damaged regions of the eye. For a successful stem cell based therapy one needs to understand the disease mechanism, determine the appropriate stem cell population, and establish/standardize the protocol for delivery/transplantation (Marchetti, et al., 2010).

The eye is divided into two anatomic regions based on the orientation from the outer surface to the inner eye contents. Cornea, conjunctiva, limbus, iris, ciliary body, and lens constitute the anterior segment, whereas the posterior segment consists of retina, choroid, and posterior sclera. Along with inflammation, the posterior segment of the eye is mostly affected with neo-vascularization and neurodegeneration, while the anterior segment is mostly affected by infection, inflammation and traumatic abrasions.

In the sections below, we discuss the localization of adult stem cells in the eye and the probable functions of stem cells based therapy, beginning from the anterior to the posterior eye segments. We have also described the potential hurdles to the success of regenerative medicine in ophthalmology.

Discussion

Cornea

The cornea - the front surface of the eye is our window to the world; hence, maintenance of corneal tissue transparency is essential for vision. The integrity and functionality of the outermost corneal layer, the epithelium, play a key role in refraction of light to the retina at the back of the eye. Like any other epithelia, the corneal epithelium is maintained by stem cells.

During development, the human cornea is one of the last ocular structures to form. Interactions between the lens vesicle and overlying surface ectoderm, as well as involvement of WNT signaling pathways and the oculogenic transcription factor Pax6, are critical for epithelial development (Davis and Piatigorsky, 2011; Nakatsu, et al., 2011; Zhang, et al., 2001). The adult cornea is a lamellar-structured tissue composed of a stratified epithelium, a collagenous substantia propria (stroma) sparsely populated with keratocytes, and an inner monolayer of endothelium, with each cell type separated by a specialized membrane, anteriorly by Bowman's layer and posteriorly by Descemet's membrane (Ordonez and Di Girolamo, 2012). The corneal stem cells preferentially express certain enzymes - for example, enolase shows an abundance of epidermal growth factor receptors, co-expresses CK 19 and vimentin, but does not express the differentiation marker, keratin K3/K12 (Dua, 1995; Dua, et al., 2003).

Identification and Isolation

Corneal epithelium is traditionally thought to be self-sufficient, self-renewing tissue. Its stem cells are located in the basal cell layer of peripheral cornea in the limbal region (Sun and Lavker, 2004).

The epithelium of the cornea contains stem cells which have the capacity to generate two different epithelial tissues: corneal and conjunctival. These cells are activated in everyday corneal renewal (Di Girolamo, 2011; Proulx, et al., 2010).

Limbal basal cells lack differentiation markers such as the 64 kDa CK3 that is present in all other layers of the corneal epithelium and the suprabasal layers of the limbal epithelium. The corneal specific 55 kD protein, CK 12, is also expressed in a similar pattern. Furthermore, connexin 43 and involucrin, both markers of cells destined for differentiation, are also absent. The transcription factor p63 is required for formation of epidermis and has been proposed as a positive limbal epithelial stem cell (LESC) marker. Limbal epithelial cells, expressing high levels of p63 with a high nuclear to cytoplasmic ratio, appear to be more stem-like. Further work has since indicated that the ΔNp63α isoform may label LESC more specifically (Chaloin-Dufau, et al., 1990; Chen, et al., 2004; Di Iorio, et al., 2005; Shortt, et al., 2007).

ABCG2 is expressed on LESCs and a few suprabasal cells. It has been proposed to be a universal marker for stem cells (Watanabe, et al., 2004; Zhou, et al., 2001). ABCG2 positive cells produce higher colony-forming efficiency values *in vitro* than their negative counterparts do (de Paiva, et al., 2005). Integrin β1 was originally suggested to be a keratinocyte marker. Limbal basal epithelial cells are described as β1 integrin bright, as are the stem cells of the epidermis, suggesting a gradient of expression that decreases with differentiation. Expression of N-cadherin in a subpopulation of limbal epithelial basal cells and in adjacent melanocytes implies that N-cadherin plays an important role in interactions between LESC and their corresponding niche cells (Hayashi, et al., 2007).

Cell clusters in the palisades of Vogt have been found with some co-localization with ABCG2 (38). Cell-cell communication is facilitated by gap junctions; hence, connexin 43 (Cx 43) and connexin 50 (Cx 50) are present in the corneal epithelium. The RNA binding protein, Musashi-1, is produced in the developing and adult eye and has recently been found in putative LESCs co-cultured with amniotic epithelial cells as feeders (Chen, et al., 2007).

Therapeutic Implication

The cornea is comprised of five layers: the outermost non-keratinized stratified epithelium, Bowman's layer, a highly ordered keratocyte-populated collagenous stroma, Descemet's membrane, and the inner endothelium (a cellular monolayer). Constant cyclic shedding and replacement or self-renewal maintain corneal integrity and ability to fulfill its refractive and protective roles (Gan, et al., 1995; Secker and Daniels, 2008a).

Stem cells found in the corneal epithelium are activated in everyday corneal renewal, whereas stem cells residing at the limbus have a different role; they are only activated when the cornea is seriously wounded. This distribution of stem cells and the different roles played by stem cells in different zones of the eye may be explained by the presence of expanding epithelia of the cornea and the conjunctiva that act like tectonic plates, squeezing the limbus between them into a kind of equilibrium zone. The limbus is already recognized as a source of cells for corneal stem-cell therapy in humans, however the cornea can also be explored as a potential source of these cells. Transient amplifying cells (TAC) compress the proliferative population of the central epithelium; this finding suggests that given appropriate signals even the TAC have flexibility of being converted to epidermis and its appendages (O'Callaghan and Daniels, 2011; Sun and Lavker, 2004).

Along with limbal stem cell deficiency, limbal dermoid, ocular surface malignancy and chronic trachoma lead to depletion of stem cells. In such cases, conjunctival phenotype invades corneal surface, where the barrier effect is lost. Conjunctivalization of cornea leads to irregular tear film, calcification, and scarring. There is evidence that normal corneal epithelium is maintained and replenished by surrounding conjunctival epithelium through the process of conjunctival transdifferentiation. Long-term observation, where partial conjunctivalization had occurred, failed to show transdifferentiation (Kinoshita, et al., 1983; Kruse, et al., 1990). Successful management of ocular surface disorders was made by conjunctival and limbal transplantation. The goal of the procedures is healing of persistent epithelial defects, reduction of corneal vascularization, improvement of vision, and patient comfort. Conjunctival transplantation was not satisfactory. Animal models have shown better results with limbal transplantation keratoepithelioplasty, a procedure wherein lamellar disc of limbal tissue, transplanted to periphery of host cornea was used in some ocular conditions such as chemical injury, Stevens-Johnson syndrome and aniridia (Amano, et al., 1992; Kaufman, 1984; Turgeon, et al., 1990; Yao, et al., 1994).

Conjunctiva

The conjunctiva is pivotal to ocular functionality as it contains essential support to cells, serves for passage of nutrients, fluids and it acts as a barrier to entry of pathogens and fluid loss. Conjunctiva consists of an epithelium covering slack and vascularized connective tissue (Du, et al., 2005).

The conjunctiva arises from a precursor into two cell types: non-keratinized, non-goblet conjunctival epithelial cells, and goblet cells (Pellegrini, et al., 1999; Wei, et al., 1997). The function of goblet cells is to produce mucin for the tear film, that is essential for ocular surface integrity, immune defense and acts as a mechanical barrier (Qi, et al., 2010). The thin transparent mucous membrane is made of a non-keratinized epithelium and a vascularized stroma. The conjunctival epithelium extends at the bulbar, fornical, and palpebral conjunctiva (Pellegrini, et al., 1999) until the mucocutaneous junction at the palpebral rim (Wirtschafter, et al., 1999).

The conjunctival epithelial cells are constantly renewed like the corneal epithelial cells. The origin of the stem cells that supply conjunctiva is not clearly defined. Studies have shown that slow-cycling ('label-retaining' cells) have been identified in the fornix (Wei, et al., 1995) and have a proliferative capacity when compared to either bulbar or palpebral conjunctival cells (Wei, et al., 1993). These studies suggest that the fornix is the stem cell niche of the conjunctival epithelium. Other related studies reveal that slow-cycling label-retaining cells are also present in the palpebral conjunctiva in rabbits as well as in rats (Chen, et al., 2003). Conjunctival stem cell biology has not been investigated as much as that of corneal stem cells (Ang, et al., 2004). Further investigation is required in order to establish the clinical implications and the role of conjunctival stem cells in ocular health.

Conjunctivalization is an overgrowth of conjunctiva on the cornea and deficiency of the limbal region called limbal stem cell deficiency (Thoft and Friend, 1983). Ocular processes that affect the cornea also affect the conjunctiva; they include scarring, cicatricial pemphigoid, adhesions, graft versus host disease, autoimmune disease, dry eye or mucin deficiency, conjunctival thickening, forniceal shortening, symblepharon, and myriad post-surgical changes, all of which affect tear film stability. When conjunctiva is required to replace diseased or damaged tissue, autografts of healthy conjunctiva can be used to generate conjunctival stem cells upon a support such as amniotic membrane (Meller, et al., 2002, Vastine, et al., 1982).

Identification and Isolation

Unlike stem cells of the corneal epithelium, conjunctival stem cells are not unipotent; they differentiate into either a mucin-secreting goblet cell or an epithelial cell (Chen, et al., 2003; Wei, et al., 1995). The basal mitotic cells from bulbar conjunctiva migrate to the surface, become quiescent as they differentiate, but do not undergo a lateral migration such as those in the cornea. The surface of cell markers expression also differs from corneal epithelium. Cornea is positive for CK3, CK12, whereas conjunctiva is positive for CK19 and cytokeratin markers. Clonal culture assays give rise to both epithelial cells and goblet cells in fornix region. These studies support the idea of a stem cell population in a fornical niche (Besharse, et al., 2010; Dua, 1995).

Therapeutic Implication

Similar to limbal auto grafts, oral mucous membrane grafts having amniotic membrane are used for conjunctival scarring. For long term success, transplanted tissue must have epithelial stem cells (Pellegrini, et al., 1999).

Limbus

The surface of the eye is covered by two distinct epithelial populations, the conjunctival and the corneal epithelium. Stem cell population for the corneal epithelium has been found to be located at the area known as the limbus. Corneal epithelial cells residing in the limbus are known as limbal epithelial stem cells (LESCs). These cells were initially identified based on an observation that the pigmented epithelium migrated in circles from limbus to central cornea during healing of epithelial defects (Secker and Daniels, 2008b).

This stem cell population is responsible for generating transient amplifying cells, which in turn are responsible for renewing the corneal epithelial cells (Ebrahimi, et al., 2009; O'Sullivan and Clynes, 2007). LESCs share common features with other adult somatic stem cells including small size (Ebrahimi, et al., 2009; Romano, et al., 2003) and high nuclear to cytoplasmic ratio (Barrandon and Green, 1987). They also lack expression of differentiation markers, "negative limbal basal cell markers" such as cytokeratins 3 and 12. Positive limbal basal cell markers characterize with expression of PAX6, p63 α and keratin 19. LESCs are slow cycling during homeostasis and therefore retain DNA labels for long time periods; however, in the event of injury they can become highly proliferative (Cotsarelis, et al., 1989; Daniels, et al., 2007; Ebrahimi, et al., 2009; Fatima, et al., 2007; Lavker, et al., 1991; Mariappan, et al., 2010; Notara, et al., 2007). To replenish the stem cell pool, stem cells have the ability to divide asymmetrically giving rise to corneal epithelial cells. Clinical evidence also points toward the limbus as a depository for a stem cell population. During homeostasis, the limbal epithelial cells are thought to act as a barrier preventing conjunctival epithelial cells from encroaching upon the cornea (Lehrer, et al., 1998; O'Callaghan and Daniels, 2011; Tseng, 1989). During LESC failure, the conjunctiva can invade the cornea causing chronic inflammation, painful corneal opacity, and neovascularization.

Identification and Isolation

Limbus harbors corneal adult stem cells. Adult stem cells are believed to reside in anatomical structures known as crypts or niches which protect their "stem cellness" by receiving various short and long range signals that control cell fate (Ordonez and Di Girolamo, 2012; Osei-Bempong, et al., 2012; Pellegrini, et al., 1999; Potten and Loeffler, 1990; Vemuganti, et al., 2009). LESCs are located within the basal interpalisade epithelial papillae of the *Palisades of Vogt* and are often visualized in small clusters. The stromal matrix and basement membrane of the ridges are closely associated with LESCs, enabling them to communicate through cell-to-cell, cell-to-ECM, or paracrine signals. Furthermore, the depth of the epithelial–stromal papillae may shelter stem cells (SCs) from physical shearing stressors, while the palisades provide a larger surface area to accommodate more SCs within a confined zone. Areas of limbus abundant in crypts and stromal projections also contain cells expressing LESC markers. The corneal epithelial basal cell population appears more differentiated than other epithelial basal cell populations, because corneal epithelial basal cells consist solely of transient amplifying cells with varying degrees of maturity as a heterogenous layer

(O'Sullivan and Clynes, 2007; Ordonez and Di Girolamo, 2012; Osei-Bempong, et al., 2012). The basement membrane beneath the LESC harbors growth factors and cytokines to regulate LESC function. The oxygen tension in the LESC niche also dictates the maintenance of limbal epithelial colonies and of the undifferentiated state of the cells (Miyashita, et al., 2007; O'Callaghan, et al., 2011).

The ability to identify stem cells (SCs) in different organs has been hampered by unreliable and nonspecific markers. The ATP-binding cassette protein (ABC) G2 is a cell surface transporter protein thought to protect LESCs from oxidative stress induced by toxins (Meyer-Blazejewska, et al., 2010; Qi, et al., 2010; Vasania, et al., 2011). ABCG2 supports progenitors by transporting small regulatory molecules required for their proliferation, differentiation, and apoptosis. Side population cells are visualized by flow cytometry and commonly include SCs that are able to efflux the fluorescent dye Hoechst 33342. ABCG2 is responsible for effluxing this dye from side population cells and the presence of these cells within the limbus correlates with ABCG2 expression. The transcription factor p63 is important for epithelial development and has been used to distinguish SCs from their transient amplifying cells (TAC) progeny in the cornea. Only the ΔNp63α isoform has been shown to be highly expressed in the limbus during resting state, whereas in the cornea, it is undetectable (Ainscough, et al., 2011; Chen, et al., 2007; O'Sullivan and Clynes, 2007; Vasania, et al., 2011). p63α /ABCG2 cells display morphological and functional features of LESCs. N-Cadherin and cytokeratin-15 are two other promising candidate LESC antigens, which colocalize to clusters of progenitor-like cells in the limbus. Resting stem cells and early transiently amplifying cells are believed to express ΔNp63α, although a counter view states that only true limbal stem cells express ΔNp63α when stimulated (Schermer, et al., 1986; Shortt, et al., 2008; Stepp, et al., 1995). Immunohistochemical analysis consistently reveals the presence of the differentiated marker cytokeratin (CK) 3 in the epithelium of limbal cornea and in the suprabasal cells of limbus, but not in the basal epithelium, suggesting the primitive nature of the basal cell. Clusters of cells expressing the integrin α9 have been localized in the basal epithelium of the limbus (Echevarria and Di Girolamo, 2011; Schermer, et al., 1986; Stepp, et al., 1995).

The microenvironment of the limbus differs from that of the central cornea by the presence and close proximity of blood vessels to the basal epithelial cells. The basement membrane of the limbus is modified to enhance epithelial cell adhesion and possesses an abundance of type IV collagen, which is absent in the central cornea (Li, et al., 2005; Ljubimov, et al., 1995; Secker and Daniels, 2008a).

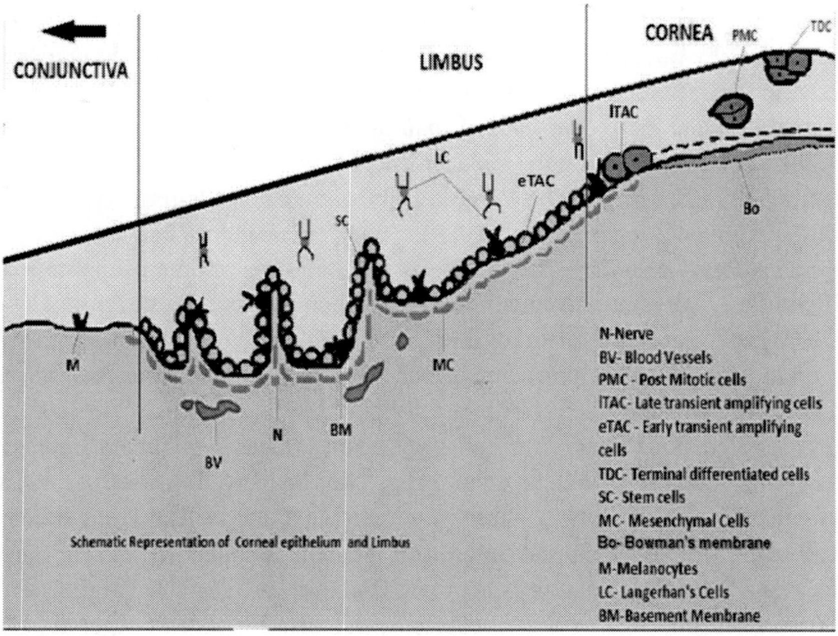

Figure 1. Schematic representation of limbal epithelial cells.

Therapeutic Implication

The ocular surface is exposed to the environment and has a constant turnover of cells to maintain the optical transparency of the cornea. These cells are regenerated from reserved LESCs, which are found at the limbus. The function of limbal stem cells is to regenerate the epithelial surface of cornea, while serving as a barrier between conjunctiva and cornea, thereby preventing loss of corneal transparency (Daniels, et al., 2007; Sangwan, et al., 2011; Sangwan, et al., 2006; Sangwan, et al., 2003; Secker and Daniels, 2008b). This property of LESCs is harnessed for limbal epithelial transplantation. Limbal epithelial stem cell deficiency is characterized by damaged or dysfunctional limbal stem cells with invasion of conjunctival epithelium onto the cornea as main features of disease. As a consequence, patients suffer from recurrent epithelial defects, persistent pain from continuous breakdown of ocular surface integrity, and inflammation (Dua, et al., 2000). LESC deficiency can occur because of primary or acquired injury. Partial or full LESC deficiency leads to deleterious effects on corneal wound healing and surface integrity. Primary injuries include mechanical, chemical or thermal burns. Acquired LESC deficiency can occur in diseases such as aniridia and Stevens Johnson syndrome. Because of LESC deficiency, conjunctivalization, neovascularization, chronic inflammation, recurrent erosions, ulceration, and stromal scarring can occur causing painful vision loss. Long-term restoration of visual function through replacement of the stem cell population has traditionally been achieved by grafting limbal auto- or allografts (Chen, et al., 2007; Kenyon and Tseng, 1989). Each procedure carries risks for complications or inducing side effects of long-term immunosuppression in allografts. As an alternative, cultured LESC therapy has been developed where LESCs are expanded *in vitro* for therapeutic application in patients in a variety of protocols utilizing amniotic membrane or fibrin, in the presence or absence of growth arrested 3T3 fibroblast feeder layers. Recently, it has been demonstrated that other stem cell populations, including human embryonic stem cells and hair follicle stem cells, can be driven towards a corneal epithelial-like phenotype. These exciting data may lead to alternative therapeutic strategies in the future for patients blinded by ocular surface diseases caused by LESC dysfunction (Chen, et al., 2007; Pellegrini, et al., 2007; Pellegrini, et al., 1999; Secker and Daniels, 2008b; Shortt, et al., 2008; Varghese, et al., 2010).

Aniridia represents a spectrum of conditions including iris anatomy defects ranging from total absence of iris to mild stomal hypoplasia with a pupil of normal appearance. Aniridic-related keratopathy (ARK) is the leading cause of progressive blindness in these patients and the LESC deficiency is most probably the underlying pathology of ARK (Mackman, et al., 1979).

Treatment for these patients involves replacement of LESC, either by keratolimbal allografts or by more recently *ex vivo* expanded LESC grafts. Patients who receive both limbal and corneal transplantation tissue seem to have a better outcome, suggesting an abnormality in the corneal tissue as well as in the limbus (Daniels, et al., 2007; Mackman, et al., 1979; Secker and Daniels, 2008b; Shortt, et al., 2008).

Iris

The two layers of epithelium derive from the marginal region of the optic cup (neuroectoderm). Sphincter and dilator pupillae muscles derive from the anterior epithelium (neuroectoderm). Stroma and blood vessels of the iris develop from the vascular mesenchyme at the anterior of to the optic cup. Iris divides the space between the cornea and lens into anterior and posterior chambers (Grierson, et al., 2002; Nita, et al., 2012).

Identification and Isolation

Iris pigment epithelial cells can be grown *in vitro* in spheres that express markers for neural stem/progenitor cells. These cells from the spheres stain for neural stem cell markers such as Nestin, Msi and Pax6. Neuronal and glial differentiation markers such as Chx10, Rho, Otx2, and Olig2 are also expressed. Cells isolated from the iris epithelium of the mouse could be differentiated into retinal neurons in the presence of guidance cue in the culture medium (Aoki, et al., 2008; Arnhold, et al., 2004; Asami, et al., 2007; Sun, et al., 2006; Wohl, et al., 2012).

Therapeutic Implication

The above mentioned studies suggest that stem cells from the iris epithelium have all the necessary attributes to repair damaged retina, however further research is needed to prove this hypothesis. Iris pigment epithelium cells from adult murine eyes have shown potential to transdifferentiate into retinal neurons *in vitro* and to express retinal specific antigens. However, there is a lack of understanding concerning long-term cell survival and stem cell properties of isolated cells (Seko, et al., 2012; Sun, et al., 2006).

Ciliary Body

The ciliary body is a forward continuation of the choroid at ora serrata. The two layers of ciliary epithelium develop from the anterior part of the two layers of the optic cup (neuroectoderm). The ciliary body stroma, ciliary muscle, and blood vessels develop from the vascular layer of the mesenchyme surrounding the optic cup. Each processus is lined by two layers of epithelial cells. The core of the ciliary processus contains blood vessels and loose connective tissue.

The ciliary processes are the site of aqueous production. The ciliary body is not only a site of aqueous humor production, but also a multifunctional organ involved in controll of aqueous humor inflow and outflow, regulation of ciliary blood flow, maintenance of the immune privilege status of the anterior chamber and of the intraocular pressure (Napier and Kidson, 2007). Until now, the role of retinal stem cells in the ciliary body remains unclear. Whether proliferative cells are involved in the above regulations is still an unresolved issue (Wohl, et al., 2012).

Cells from the ciliary body, but not the sensory neural retina, have been shown to generate neurospheres that express nestin, a marker for somatic neural progenitor cells (Tropepe, et al., 2000). The number of neurospheres generated from both the iris and the pars plana was 2–3 times greater than that isolated from the ciliary body, suggesting that these regions may be particularly rich in stem/progenitor cells. Individual neurospheres from each of the three regions were similar in size, indicating that they have comparable expansion potential when grown as neurospheres (Jasty, et al., 2012; MacNeil, et al., 2007).

Identification and Isolation

Ciliary body stem cells arise from the ciliary epithelium and have neurogenic potential.

The expression of Chx10 and Pax6 can be taken as evidence that ciliary-derived progenitors have potential to develope into retinal tissues. Other investigators have reported the expression of mature retinal cell markers in ciliary progenitors (Tsonis and Fuentes, 2006).

In addition to expressing stem or progenitor markers, such as nestin, ciliary progenitors also express vimentin. Ki-67 provide more specific evidence of the course of cell division; ciliary progenitor cells have been reported to express homeobox genes that are prominent in normal retinal development, including Chx10 and Pax6 (Ahmad, et al., 2004; Reh and Levine, 1998).

Ciliary epithelial cells that are cultured *in vitro* form both neurosphere and monolayer. These cultures express the developmentally regulated transcription factors Sox2 and Pax 6 together with retinal markers including Lhx2, Dach1, and Six3 (Xu, et al., 2007).

Therapeutic Implication

Neurospheres derived from the ciliary epithelium may be potential sources of adult progenitor cells, capable of differentiating into neural phenotypes. Studies have demonstrated that neurospheres containing progenitor cells could derive not only from the ciliary body but also from the iris and pars plana. Moreover, these cells could form retinal neuronal cells, as well as glial cell types.

In normal conditions, the cells from the ciliary epithelium maintain a balance between the epithelial and the neuronal cell types in the eye by transdifferentiation. In pathological conditions, these cells from the ciliary epithelium may act as donor cells for retinal repair (Gu, et al., 2007; Xu, et al., 2007; Yanagi, et al., 2006).

Several attempts have been made to differentiate ciliary epithelial cells into retinal neurons in order to repair the damaged retina. The results so far have revealed that the integration is unstable, although the differentiated retinal cells express all the markers for retinal cells.

Lens

Lens is a component of the anterior chamber of the eye that refracts and directs light to be focused on the retina for the perception of image. Lens is composed of lens capsule, epithelium, and fibers.

Lens stem cells have not been identified so far. It is hypothesized that lental stem cells are residing outside the lens capsule. Ciliary body might be the plausible source of lental stem cells regarding its proximity to the lens (Remington and Meyer, 2007). Studies including lower vertebrates have revealed regeneration of lens from cells residing in the ciliary body (Stone, 1965; Tsonis and Del Rio-Tsonis, 2004).

Therapeutic Implication

Lens progenitors derive from human embryonic stem cells and from other induced pluripotent stem cells by differentiation, as well as by transdifferentiation (Qiu, et al., 2012; Yang, et al., 2010). Lental stem cells have yet to be identified. Their therapeutic implications could be associated primarily with cataractogenesis and other lens abnormalities.

Retina

The cornea and the retina represent the most important future promising areas for ocular stem cell treatment. The easy access to the cornea, the homologous of corneal epithelium forming different layers and the improvement of protocols are considerable alleviations in corneal epithelium restorations. Likewise, retinal restoration has been achieved in various animal models using photoreceptors, transplantation of endothelial cells, and retinal pigment epithelium (RPE) cells (Pellegrini, et al., 2007).

Diseases, pertaining to the posterior region of the eye involving retinal neurons, retinal pigment epithelium or retinal vasculature, such as inherited retinal degenerations, age-related macular degeneration, diabetic retinopathy, retinopathy of prematurity etc., are more challenging to treat with cell-based therapy. Several attempts have been made for treating these conditions using cell-based therapy (Meyer, et al., 2011; Rowland, et al., 2012).

Therapeutic Implication

Several studies reported achievement of visual function by transplantation of cells in a rat model of retinal degeneration; however, the level of function of the existing photoreceptors is unclear (Sagdullaev, et al., 2003; Seiler and Aramant, 2005; Seiler, et al., 1999). Nevertheless, the studies suggested that grafting might be an accepted therapeutic strategy for retinal degenerations.

MacLaren et al (2006) reported that donor cells can integrate into an adult or degenerated retina if they are taken from the developing retina at a time coincident with the peak of rod genesis.

These transplanted cells integrate, differentiate into rod photoreceptors, form synaptic connections and improve visual function. Small clinical trials had been attempted using fetal retinal cells containing RPE (Radtke, et al., 2004; Radtke, et al., 2002), retinal aggregates (Das, et al., 1999; Humayun, et al., 2000), or adult retinal sheets (Kaplan, et al., 1997) in patients suffering from retinitis pigmentosa and age-related macular degeneration. Human tissues are limited sources and stem cells could be an alternative for transplantation. The above mentioned studies show promising outcomes regarding transplantation for the repair of damaged retinal cells (Pellegrini, et al., 2007).

Retinal-Pigmented Epithelium

Stem cell–based therapy is related with various procedures that involve both the cellular/extracellular matrix microenvironment into which stem cells are injected (Blazejewska, et al., 2009). The injected stem cells integrate to retinal and sub-retinal micro environment that modulate differentiation of different cell types (Banin, et al., 2006; Kustermann, et al., 2010; MacLaren, et al., 2006). Small molecules can be incorporated or conjugated with stem cells before transplantation to make specific differentiation pathways (MacLaren, et al., 2006). These cells serve to replace the damaged cells and produce cytokines, growth factors, and other trophic molecules (Sengupta, et al., 2009). The current stem cell–based therapies for retinal diseases focus on supplementing or replacing photoreceptors and RPE in the affected retina (Marchetti, et al., 2010).

Therapeutic Implication

The initial results of clinical trials of subretinal transplantation of human embryonic stem cell-derived retinal pigment epithelium cells in patients with Stargardt's macular dystrophy and dry age-related macular degeneration showed preliminary safety and possible visual acuity benefits (Tibbetts, et al., 2012). Under good manufacturing practices approved by US food and drug administration (FDA), human embryonic stem cells (hESCs) were derived into RPE and transplanted into a rat model of retinal degeneration (Lu, et al., 2009). Long-term data (spanning the life of the animals) showed no gross or microscopic evidence of teratoma/tumor formation after subretinal hESC-RPE transplantation. Usually the yield of RPE from ESCs is less than 1%, but recent work has much developed to give rise of 33% in addition of vitamin B3 and activin A protein for cell differentiation (Idelson, et al., 2009). Protocols had been published in detailed manner about mouse and human ESCs into photoreceptors (Lamba, et al., 2006; Osakada, et al., 2009). Human ESCs were differentiated into retinal precursors and transplanted into sub-retinal space and they restored partial light sensitivity without causing teratoma in the rat model of Leber's congenital amaurosis (Lamba, et al., 2009).

Replacement of RPE in age-related macular degeneration (AMD) has been studied in clinical trials (Algvere, et al., 1999; Peyman, et al., 1991; Weisz, et al., 1999). The acquired vision after the procedure had been transient (MacLaren, et al., 2005; Stanga, et al., 2002). Transplantation of autologous RPE revealed better results (Binder, et al., 2004). The major technical hurdle of the procedure was in harvesting healthy RPE to generate cell lines. However, cultured RPE cells were first transplanted in a Royal College Surgeon (RCS) rat model of AMD, which had a mutation in Mertk gene leading to the loss of phagocytosis ability of the RPE cells that resulted in accumulation of photoreceptors (D'Cruz, et al., 2000; Nandrot, et al., 2000). AMD studies that used that model indicate that transplanted rodent RPE cells eliminate photoreceptor debris and maintain visual function in the transplanted retinal area (Lund, et al., 2001).

Currently, rather than replacing single cells, the entire retina is replaced with differentiated stem cells (Ali and Sowden, 2011). The three-dimensional neural retina was grown in culture from mouse ESCs (Eiraku, et al., 2011). ESCs were cultured with extracellular matrix and had undergone morphogenesis to develop bilayered cups. These cups visibly pigmented and expressed molecular markers of neural retina and RPE. They can be further differentiated into photoreceptors and can be used for testing in pharmacology and other therapies.

Clinical trials are carried out for retinal diseases like Stargardt's macular dystrophy and geographic atrophy in AMD using RPE derived from ESCs. There have been preliminary reports on transplantation of RPE cells derived from ESC into patients having Stargardt's macular dystrophy and geographic atrophy in AMD using sub-retinal injections. Before transplantation, the culture was studied extensively for purity and pathogenicity (Schwartz, et al., 2012). Further studies are necessary for the utilization of RPE transplantation into a human, so that these cells can be integrated effectively in the retina while being free of malignancy and immunogenicity (Lakowski, et al., 2011; Lamba, et al., 2010). Immune suppression of recipients significantly increased transplanted photoreceptor survival (West, et al., 2010).

Choroid

The term *choroid* is derived from the Greek words for "*membrane*" and "*form*"; the choriocapillaris was first described by Hovius in 1702, and named in 1838 by Eschricht (Abdouh and Bernier, 2006). The choroid derives from mesoderm and neuroectoderm (Booij, et al., 2010).

There are sparse reports of the presence of mesenchymal stem cells in choroid of murines (Kivela and Uusitalo, 1998; Tsai, et al., 2011). Not much is known or investigated in the differentiation potential as well as of the self-renewal attributes of these cells. These cells obtained from mouse tissue were positive for the mesenchymal markers Sca-1, CD90.2, CD44, CD105, and CD73 and negative for the hematopoietic markers. Additionally the isolated cells expressed stem cell markers such as ABCG2, Six2, Notch1, and Pax6.

Therapeutic Implication

Future studies are needed to identify stem cells in the choroid of humans. All the studies to date have reported the presence of such cells only in murine species.

These cells might play a pivotal role in the neurodegenerative ocular diseases. Scleral as well as choroidal cells from adult human eyes were differentiated to retinal neurons in laboratories. Not much is understood about their long-term survival potential, although the differentiated cells expressed retinal antigens (Arsenijevic, et al., 2003; Mullins, et al., 2012). Further studies are needed for these cells to be used in treatment.

Sclera

Sclera maintains the shape of the eye and it is composed of fibrous material. It is in continuation with the cornea and has four layers: episclera, stroma, lamina fusca and endothelium (Keeley, et al., 1984). Scleral stem cells have been identified in mouse sclera. The isolated stem cells are of mesenchymal origin and have all the classical properties of stem/progenitor cells. Scleral stem cells express the pluripotent markers: ABCG2, Six2, Pax 6, and Notch1 (Tsai, et al., 2011).

Therapeutic Implication

Scleral diseases often lead to blindness because of lack of proper cure. If identified, scleral stem cells may be able to provide some mode of treatment for diseases such as scleritis and scleromalacia. Human scleral tissue has chondrogenic potential and could be used for treating patients with rheumatoid diseases. Diseases such as myopia might be related to scleral distension, which might be repaired using the scleral stem/progenitor cells. These cells may also provide vital clues for synthesizing artificial sclera, which would have implications in conditions involving the shape of eye as an oculoplastic tool.

Conclusion

In this review, we attempted to address all the known sources of stem cells in the adult eye and their potentials for cell replacement as a therapeutic tool. Stem cell based therapy is an emerging field that is visualized as a panacea for all vascular and neurodegenerative diseases of the eye. Identifying the cells and characterizing them well is just the first step in the long journey of stem cell based treatment. Ophthalmology has been privileged to be the first field of medical science where stem cell treatment has been widely approved (limbal epithelial stem cell transplantation). Another important aspect of using stem cell treatment would be the stage of a disease; that is, in neurodegenerative diseases early intervention is the only possible way to cure or prevent the progress of retinal-neuronal network damage. For successful utilization of the stem cells for therapeutic purposes, the basic researchers need to unravel the role of the "ivy league" signaling pathways such as Notch, WNT, Jak-Stat, Tyrosine kinase, Sonic hedge-hog (Das, et al., 2010; Liu, et al., 2011). Future basic and clinical research are expected to provide valuable information regarding the potential of these cells for treatment in various ophthalmic pathology.

Stem cell based therapy provides a major hope for the restoration of sight in blind patients where the vision is lost by irreversible damage caused by a disease or trauma. There is a lot of speculation concerning ocular stem cells and their potential to de-differentiate or transdifferentiate to cell types of our interest. Before taking a big step in clinics, we need to establish protocols for identification/isolation, as well as differentiation of ocular stem cells. There seem to be some hurdles in the technicality, but there is enough optimism among basic researchers as well as ophthalmologists worldwide to make stem cell based therapies a reality.

Acknowledgments

The authors would like to thank Dr. K Bhujang Shetty and Dr. Rohit Shetty for providing all the necessary logistics and support for the completion of this chapter.

References

Abdouh, M., and Bernier, G. (2006). In vivo reactivation of a quiescent cell population located in the ocular ciliary body of adult mammals. *Exp. Eye Res.* 83(1): 153-164.

Ahmad, I., Das, A. V., James, J., Bhattacharya, S., and Zhao, X. (2004). Neural stem cells in the mammalian eye: types and regulation. *Semin. Cell. Dev. Biol.* 15(1): 53-62.

Ainscough, S. L., Linn, M. L., Barnard, Z., Schwab, I. R., and Harkin, D. G. (2011). Effects of fibroblast origin and phenotype on the proliferative potential of limbal epithelial progenitor cells. *Exp Eye Res.* 92(1): 10-19.

Algvere, P. V., Gouras, P., and Dafgard Kopp, E. (1999). Long-term outcome of RPE allografts in non-immunosuppressed patients with AMD. *Eur. J. Ophthalmo.* 9(3): 217-230.

Ali, R. R., and Sowden, J. C. (2011). Regenerative medicine: DIY eye. *Nature.* 472 (7341): 42-43.

Amano, S., Sawa, M., and Ishii, Y. (1992). Keratoepithelioplasty in rat: development of a model and histological study. *Jpn. J. Ophthalmol.* 36(4): 407-416.

Ang, L. P., Tan, D. T., Beuerman, R. W., and Lavker, R. M. (2004). Development of a conjunctival epithelial equivalent with improved proliferative properties using a multistep serum-free culture system. *Invest. Ophthalmol. Vis. Sci.* 45(6):1789-1795.

Aoki, H., Hara, A., Motohashi, T., Chem, H., and Kunisada, T. (2008). Iris as a recipient tissue for pigment cells: organized in vivo differentiation of melanocytes and pigmented epithelium derived from embryonic stem cells in vitro. *Dev. Dyn.* 237(9): 2394-2404.

Arnhold, S., Semkova, I., Andressen, C., Lenartz, D., Meissner, G., Sturm, V., et al. (2004). Iris pigment epithelial cells: a possible cell source for the future treatment of neurodegenerative diseases. *Exp. Neurol.* 187(2): 410-417.

Arsenijevic, Y., Taverney, N., Kostic, C., Tekaya, M., Riva, F., Zografos, L., et al. (2003). Non-neural regions of the adult human eye: a potential source of neurons? *Invest. Ophthalmol. Vis. Sci.* 44(2): 799-807.

Asami, M., Sun, G., Yamaguchi, M., and Kosaka, M. (2007). Multipotent cells from mammalian iris pigment epithelium. *Dev Biol.* 304(1): 433-446.

Banin, E., Obolensky, A., Idelson, M., Hemo, I., Reinhardtz, E., Pikarsky, E., et al. (2006). Retinal incorporation and differentiation of neural precursors derived from human embryonic stem cells. *Stem Cells.* 24(2): 246-257.

Barrandon, Y., and Green, H. (1987). Three clonal types of keratinocyte with different capacities for multiplication. *Proc. Natl. Acad. Sci. U S A.* 84(8): 2302-2306.

Besharse, J., Dana, R., and Dartt, D. A. (2010). *Encyclopedia of the Eye Online*: Elsevier Science.

Binder, S., Krebs, I., Hilgers, R. D., Abri, A., Stolba, U., Assadoulina, A., et al. (2004). Outcome of transplantation of autologous retinal pigment epithelium in age-related macular degeneration: a prospective trial. *Invest. Ophthalmol. Vis. Sci.* 45(11): 4151-4160.

Blazejewska, E. A., Schlotzer-Schrehardt, U., Zenkel, M., Bachmann, B., Chankiewitz, E., Jacobi, C., et al. (2009). Corneal limbal microenvironment can induce transdifferentiation of hair follicle stem cells into corneal epithelial-like cells. *Stem. Cells.* 27(3):642-652.

Booij, J. C., Baas, D. C., Beisekeeva, J., Gorgels, T. G., and Bergen, A. A. (2010). The dynamic nature of Bruch's membrane. *Prog. Retin. Eye Res.* 29(1): 1-18.

Chaloin-Dufau, C., Sun, T. T., and Dhouailly, D. (1990). Appearance of the keratin pair K3/K12 during embryonic and adult corneal epithelial differentiation in the chick and in the rabbit. *Cell. Differ. Dev.* 32(2): 97-108.

Chen, W., Ishikawa, M., Yamaki, K., and Sakuragi, S. (2003). Wistar rat palpebral conjunctiva contains more slow-cycling stem cells that have larger proliferative capacity: implication for conjunctival epithelial homeostasis. *Jpn. J. Ophthalmol.* 47(2): 119-128.

Chen, Y. T., Li, W., Hayashida, Y., He, H., Chen, S. Y., Tseng, D. Y., et al. (2007). Human amniotic epithelial cells as novel feeder layers for promoting ex vivo expansion of limbal epithelial progenitor cells. *Stem. Cells.* 25(8): 1995-2005.

Chen, Z., de Paiva, C. S., Luo, L., Kretzer, F. L., Pflugfelder, S. C., and Li, D. Q. (2004). Characterization of putative stem cell phenotype in human limbal epithelia. *Stem. Cells.* 22(3): 355-366.

Cotsarelis, G., Cheng, S. Z., Dong, G., Sun, T. T., and Lavker, R. M. (1989). Existence of slow-cycling limbal epithelial basal cells that can be preferentially stimulated to proliferate: implications on epithelial stem cells. *Cell.* 57(2): 201-209.

D'Cruz, P. M., Yasumura, D., Weir, J., Matthes, M. T., Abderrahim, H., LaVail, M. M., et al. (2000). Mutation of the receptor tyrosine kinase gene Mertk in the retinal dystrophic RCS rat. *Hum Mol Genet.* 9(4): 645-651.

Daniels, J. T., Notara, M., Shortt, A. J., Secker, G., Harris, A., and Tuft, S. J. (2007). Limbal epithelial stem cell therapy. *Expert. Opin. Biol. Ther.* 7(1): 1-3.

Das, D., Lanner, F., Main, H., Andersson, E. R., Bergmann, O., Sahlgren, C., et al. (2010). Notch induces cyclin-D1-dependent proliferation during a specific temporal window of neural differentiation in ES cells. *Dev. Biol.* 348(2):153-166.

Das, T., del Cerro, M., Jalali, S., Rao, V. S., Gullapalli, V. K., Little, C., et al. (1999). The transplantation of human fetal neuroretinal cells in advanced retinitis pigmentosa patients: results of a long-term safety study. *Exp. Neurol.* 157(1): 58-68.

Davis, J., and Piatigorsky, J. (2011). Overexpression of Pax6 in mouse cornea directly alters corneal epithelial cells: changes in immune function, vascularization, and differentiation. *Invest. Ophthalmol. Vis. Sci.* 52(7):4158-4168.

de Paiva, C. S., Chen, Z., Corrales, R. M., Pflugfelder, S. C., and Li, D. Q. (2005). ABCG2 transporter identifies a population of clonogenic human limbal epithelial cells. *Stem Cells.* 23(1): 63-73.

Di Girolamo, N. (2011). Stem cells of the human cornea. *Br Med Bull.* 100: 191-207.

Di Iorio, E., Barbaro, V., Ruzza, A., Ponzin, D., Pellegrini, G., and De Luca, M. (2005). Isoforms of DeltaNp63 and the migration of ocular limbal cells in human corneal regeneration. *Proc. Natl. Acad. Sci. U S A.* 102(27): 9523-9528.

Du, Y., Funderburgh, M. L., Mann, M. M., Sundar Raj, N., and Funderburgh, J. L. (2005). Multipotent stem cells in human corneal stroma. *Stem. Cells.* 23(9): 1266-1275.

Dua, H. S. (1995). Stem cells of the ocular surface: scientific principles and clinical applications. *Br. J. Ophthalmol.* 79(11): 968-969.

Dua, H. S., Joseph, A., Shanmuganathan, V. A., and Jones, R. E. (2003). Stem cell differentiation and the effects of deficiency. *Eye (Lond).* 17(8): 877-885.

Dua, H. S., Saini, J. S., Azuara-Blanco, A., and Gupta, P. (2000). Limbal stem cell deficiency: concept, aetiology, clinical presentation, diagnosis, and management. *Indian J. Ophthalmol.* 48(2):83-92.

Ebrahimi, M., Taghi-Abadi, E., and Baharvand, H. (2009). Limbal stem cells in review. *J. Ophthalmic. Vis. Res.* 4(1): 40-58.

Echevarria, T. J., and Di Girolamo, N. (2011). Tissue-regenerating, vision-restoring corneal epithelial stem cells. *Stem. Cell. Rev.* 7(2): 256-268.

Eiraku, M., Takata, N., Ishibashi, H., Kawada, M., Sakakura, E., Okuda, S., et al. (2011). Self-organizing optic-cup morphogenesis in three-dimensional culture. *Nature.* 472(7341): 51-56.

Fatima, A., Vemuganti, G. K., Iftekhar, G., Rao, G. N., and Sangwan, V. S. (2007). In vivo survival and stratification of cultured limbal epithelium. *Clin. Experiment. Ophthalmol.* 35(1):96-98.

Gan, L., van Setten, G., Seregard, S., and Fagerholm, P. (1995). Proliferating cell nuclear antigen colocalization with corneal epithelial stem cells and involvement in physiological cell turnover. *Acta. Ophthalmol. Scand.* 73(6): 491-495.

Grierson, I., Pfeiffer, N., Cracknell, K. P., and Appleton, P. (2002). Histology and fine structure of the iris and outflow system following latanoprost therapy. *Surv. Ophthalmol.* 47 Suppl 1: S176-184.

Gu, P., Harwood, L. J., Zhang, X., Wylie, M., Curry, W. J., and Cogliati, T. (2007). Isolation of retinal progenitor and stem cells from the porcine eye. *Mol. Vis.* 13: 1045-1057.

Hayashi, R., Yamato, M., Sugiyama, H., Sumide, T., Yang, J., Okano, T., et al. (2007). N-Cadherin is expressed by putative stem/progenitor cells and melanocytes in the human limbal epithelial stem cell niche. *Stem. Cells.* 25(2) :289-296.

Humayun, M. S., de Juan, E., Jr., del Cerro, M., Dagnelie, G., Radner, W., Sadda, S. R., et al. (2000). Human neural retinal transplantation. *Invest. Ophthalmol. Vis. Sci.* 41(10): 3100-3106.

Idelson, M., Alper, R., Obolensky, A., Ben-Shushan, E., Hemo, I., Yachimovich-Cohen, N., et al. (2009). Directed differentiation of human embryonic stem cells into functional retinal pigment epithelium cells. *Cell Stem. Cell.* 5(4) :396-408.

Jasty, S., Srinivasan, P., Pasricha, G., Chatterjee, N., and Subramanian, K. (2012). Gene expression profiles and retinal potential of stem/progenitor cells derived from human iris and ciliary pigment epithelium. *Stem. Cell. Rev.* 8(4): 1163-1177.

Kaplan, H. J., Tezel, T. H., Berger, A. S., Wolf, M. L., and Del Priore, L. V. (1997). Human photoreceptor transplantation in retinitis pigmentosa. A safety study. *Arch. Ophthalmol.* 115(9): 1168-1172.

Kaufman, H. E. (1984). Keratoepithelioplasty for the replacement of damaged corneal epithelium. *Am. J. Ophthalmol.* 97(1): 100-101.

Keeley, F. W., Morin, J. D., and Vesely, S. (1984). Characterization of collagen from normal human sclera. *Exp. Eye Res.* 39(5): 533-542.

Kenyon, K. R., and Tseng, S. C. (1989). Limbal autograft transplantation for ocular surface disorders. *Ophthalmology.* 96(5): 709-722; discussion 722-703.

Kinoshita, S., Friend, J., and Thoft, R. A. (1983). Biphasic cell proliferation in transdifferentiation of conjunctival to corneal epithelium in rabbits. *Invest. Ophthalmol. Vis. Sci.* 24(8)1008-1014.

Kivela, T., and Uusitalo, M. (1998). Structure, development, and function of cytoskeletal elements in non-neuronal cells of the human eye. *Prog. Retin. Eye Res.* 17(3):385-428.

Kruse, F. E., Chen, J. J., Tsai, R. J., and Tseng, S. C. (1990). Conjunctival transdifferentiation is due to the incomplete removal of limbal basal epithelium. *Invest. Ophthalmol. Vis. Sci.* 31(9): 1903-1913.

Kustermann, S., Hildebrandt, H., Bolz, S., Dengler, K., and Kohler, K. (2010). Genesis of rods in the zebrafish retina occurs in a microenvironment provided by polysialic acid-expressing Muller glia. *J. Comp. Neurol.* 518(5): 636-646.

Lakowski, J., Han, Y. T., Pearson, R. A., Gonzalez-Cordero, A., West, E. L., Gualdoni, S., et al. (2011). Effective transplantation of photoreceptor precursor cells selected via cell surface antigen expression. *Stem. Cells.* 29(9): 1391-1404.

Lamba, D. A., Gust, J., and Reh, T. A. (2009). Transplantation of human embryonic stem cell-derived photoreceptors restores some visual function in Crx-deficient mice. *Cell. Stem. Cell.* 4(1):73-79.

Lamba, D. A., Karl, M. O., Ware, C. B., and Reh, T. A. (2006). Efficient generation of retinal progenitor cells from human embryonic stem cells. *Proc. Natl. Acad. Sci. U S A.* 103(34): 12769-12774.

Lamba, D. A., McUsic, A., Hirata, R. K., Wang, P. R., Russell, D., and Reh, T. A. (2010). Generation, purification, and transplantation of photoreceptors derived from human induced pluripotent stem cells. *PLoS One*. 5(1): e8763.

Lavker, R. M., Dong, G., Cheng, S. Z., Kudoh, K., Cotsarelis, G., and Sun, T. T. (1991). Relative proliferative rates of limbal and corneal epithelia. Implications of corneal epithelial migration, circadian rhythm, and suprabasally located DNA-synthesizing keratinocytes. *Invest. Ophthalmol. Vis Sci.* 32(6): 1864-1875.

Lehrer, M. S., Sun, T. T., and Lavker, R. M. (1998). Strategies of epithelial repair: modulation of stem cell and transit amplifying cell proliferation. *J. Cell. Sci.* 111 (Pt 19): 2867-2875.

Li, D. Q., Chen, Z., Song, X. J., de Paiva, C. S., Kim, H. S., and Pflugfelder, S. C. (2005). Partial enrichment of a population of human limbal epithelial cells with putative stem cell properties based on collagen type IV adhesiveness. *Exp. Eye Res.* 80(4): 581-590.

Liu, L., Lanner, F., Lendahl, U., and Das, D. (2011). Numb-like and Numb differentially affect p53 and Sonic Hedgehog signaling. *Biochem. Biophys. Res. Commun.* 413(3) :426-431.

Ljubimov, A. V., Burgeson, R. E., Butkowski, R. J., Michael, A. F., Sun, T. T., and Kenney, M. C. (1995). Human corneal basement membrane heterogeneity: topographical differences in the expression of type IV collagen and laminin isoforms. *Lab. Invest.* 72(4): 461-473.

Lu, B., Malcuit, C., Wang, S., Girman, S., Francis, P., Lemieux, L., et al. (2009). Long-term safety and function of RPE from human embryonic stem cells in preclinical models of macular degeneration. *Stem. Cells.* 27(9): 2126-2135.

Lund, R. D., Kwan, A. S., Keegan, D. J., Sauve, Y., Coffey, P. J., and Lawrence, J. M. (2001). Cell transplantation as a treatment for retinal disease. *Prog. Retin. Eye Res.* 20(4): 415-449.

Mackman, G., Brightbill, F. S., and Optiz, J. M. (1979). Corneal changes in aniridia. *Am. J. Ophthalmol.* 87(4) :497-502.

MacLaren, R. E., Bird, A. C., Sathia, P. J., and Aylward, G. W. (2005). Long-term results of submacular surgery combined with macular translocation of the retinal pigment epithelium in neovascular age-related macular degeneration. *Ophthalmology.* 112(12): 2081-2087.

MacLaren, R. E., Pearson, R. A., MacNeil, A., Douglas, R. H., Salt, T. E., Akimoto, M., et al. (2006). Retinal repair by transplantation of photoreceptor precursors. *Nature.* 444(7116): 203-207.

MacNeil, A., Pearson, R. A., MacLaren, R. E., Smith, A. J., Sowden, J. C., and Ali, R. R. (2007). Comparative analysis of progenitor cells isolated from the iris, pars plana, and ciliary body of the adult porcine eye. *Stem. Cells.* 25(10): 2430-2438.

Marchetti, V., Krohne, T. U., Friedlander, D. F., and Friedlander, M. (2010). Stemming vision loss with stem cells. *J. Clin. Invest.* 120(9): 3012-3021.

Mariappan, I., Maddileti, S., Savy, S., Tiwari, S., Gaddipati, S., Fatima, A., et al. (2010). In vitro culture and expansion of human limbal epithelial cells. *Nat. Protoc.* 5(8): 1470-1479.

Meller, D., Dabul, V., and Tseng, S. C. (2002). Expansion of conjunctival epithelial progenitor cells on amniotic membrane. *Exp. Eye Res.* 74(4): 537-545.

Meyer-Blazejewska, E. A., Kruse, F. E., Bitterer, K., Meyer, C., Hofmann-Rummelt, C., Wunsch, P. H., et al. (2010). Preservation of the limbal stem cell phenotype by appropriate culture techniques. *Invest. Ophthalmol. Vis. Sci.* 51(2): 765-774.

Meyer, J. S., Howden, S. E., Wallace, K. A., Verhoeven, A. D., Wright, L. S., Capowski, E. E., et al. (2011). Optic vesicle-like structures derived from human pluripotent stem cells facilitate a customized approach to retinal disease treatment. *Stem. Cells.* 29(8): 1206-1218.

Miyashita, H., Higa, K., Kato, N., Kawakita, T., Yoshida, S., Tsubota, K., et al. (2007). Hypoxia enhances the expansion of human limbal epithelial progenitor cells in vitro. *Invest. Ophthalmol. Vis. Sci.* 48(8): 3586-3593.

Mullins, R. F., Kuehn, M. H., Radu, R. A., Enriquez, G. S., East, J. S., Schindler, E. I., et al. (2012). Autosomal recessive retinitis pigmentosa due to ABCA4 mutations: clinical, pathologic, and molecular characterization. *Invest. Ophthalmol. Vis. Sci.* 53(4): 1883-1894.

Nakatsu, M. N., Ding, Z., Ng, M. Y., Truong, T. T., Yu, F., and Deng, S. X. (2011). Wnt/beta-catenin signaling regulates proliferation of human cornea epithelial stem/progenitor cells. *Invest. Ophthalmol. Vis. Sci.* 52(7): 4734-4741.

Nandrot, E., Dufour, E. M., Provost, A. C., Pequignot, M. O., Bonnel, S., Gogat, K., et al. (2000). Homozygous deletion in the coding sequence of the c-mer gene in RCS rats unravels general mechanisms of physiological cell adhesion and apoptosis. *Neurobiol. Dis.* 7(6 Pt B) :586-599.

Napier, H. R., and Kidson, S. H. (2007). Molecular events in early development of the ciliary body: a question of folding. *Exp. Eye Res.* 84(4): 615-625.

Nita, M., Strzalka-Mrozik, B., Grzybowski, A., Romaniuk, W., and Mazurek, U. (2012). Ophthalmic transplantology: posterior segment of the eye--part II. *Med. Sci. Monit.* 18(6) RA97-103.

Notara, M., Haddow, D. B., MacNeil, S., and Daniels, J. T. (2007). A xenobiotic-free culture system for human limbal epithelial stem cells. *Regen. Med.* 2(6): 919-927.

O'Callaghan, A. R., and Daniels, J. T. (2011). Concise review: limbal epithelial stem cell therapy: controversies and challenges. *Stem. Cells.* 29(12):1923-1932.

O'Callaghan, A. R., Daniels, J. T., and Mason, C. (2011). Effect of sub-atmospheric oxygen on the culture of rabbit limbal epithelial cells. *Curr. Eye Res.* 36(8): 691-698.

O'Sullivan, F., and Clynes, M. (2007). Limbal stem cells, a review of their identification and culture for clinical use. *Cytotechnology.* 53(1-3): 101-106.

Ordonez, P., and Di Girolamo, N. (2012). Limbal epithelial stem cells: role of the niche microenvironment. *Stem. Cells.* 30(2):100-107.

Osakada, F., Ikeda, H., Sasai, Y., and Takahashi, M. (2009). Stepwise differentiation of pluripotent stem cells into retinal cells. *Nat. Protoc.* 4(6): 811-824.

Osei-Bempong, C., Figueiredo, F. C., and Lako, M. (2012). The limbal epithelium of the eye - A review of limbal stem cell biology, disease, and treatment. *Bioessays*.

Pellegrini, G., De Luca, M., and Arsenijevic, Y. (2007). Towards therapeutic application of ocular stem cells. *Semin. Cell Dev. Biol.* 18(6): 805-818.

Pellegrini, G., Golisano, O., Paterna, P., Lambiase, A., Bonini, S., Rama, P., et al. (1999). Location and clonal analysis of stem cells and their differentiated progeny in the human ocular surface. *J. Cell. Biol.* 145(4): 769-782.

Peyman, G. A., Blinder, K. J., Paris, C. L., Alturki, W., Nelson, N. C., Jr., and Desai, U. (1991). A technique for retinal pigment epithelium transplantation for age-related macular degeneration secondary to extensive subfoveal scarring. *Ophthalmic. Surg.* 22(2):102-108.

Potten, C. S., and Loeffler, M. (1990). Stem cells: attributes, cycles, spirals, pitfalls and uncertainties. Lessons for and from the crypt. *Development.* 110(4): 1001-1020.

Proulx, S., Fradette, J., Gauvin, R., Larouche, D., and Germain, L. (2010). Stem cells of the skin and cornea: their clinical applications in regenerative medicine. *Curr. Opin. Organ. Transplant.*

Qi, H., Zheng, X., Yuan, X., Pflugfelder, S. C., and Li, D. Q. (2010). Potential localization of putative stem/progenitor cells in human bulbar conjunctival epithelium. *J. Cell. Physiol.* 225(1):180-185.

Qiu, X., Yang, J., Liu, T., Jiang, Y., Le, Q., and Lu, Y. (2012). Efficient generation of lens progenitor cells from cataract patient-specific induced pluripotent stem cells. *PLoS One.* 7(3) :e32612.

Radtke, N. D., Aramant, R. B., Seiler, M. J., Petry, H. M., and Pidwell, D. (2004). Vision change after sheet transplant of fetal retina with retinal pigment epithelium to a patient with retinitis pigmentosa. *Arch. Ophthalmol.* 122(8):1159-1165.

Radtke, N. D., Seiler, M. J., Aramant, R. B., Petry, H. M., and Pidwell, D. J. (2002). Transplantation of intact sheets of fetal neural retina with its retinal pigment epithelium in retinitis pigmentosa patients. *Am. J. Ophthalmol.* 133(4): 544-550.

Reh, T. A., and Levine, E. M. (1998). Multipotential stem cells and progenitors in the vertebrate retina. *J. Neurobiol.* 36(2):206-220.

Remington, S. G., and Meyer, R. A. (2007). Lens stem cells may reside outside the lens capsule: a hypothesis. *Theor. Biol. Med. Model.* 4: 22.

Romano, A. C., Espana, E. M., Yoo, S. H., Budak, M. T., Wolosin, J. M., and Tseng, S. C. (2003). Different cell sizes in human limbal and central corneal basal epithelia measured by confocal microscopy and flow cytometry. *Invest. Ophthalmol. Vis. Sci.* 44(12):5125-5129.

Rowland, T. J., Buchholz, D. E., and Clegg, D. O. (2012). Pluripotent human stem cells for the treatment of retinal disease. *J. Cell Physiol.* 227(2) :457-466.

Sagdullaev, B. T., Aramant, R. B., Seiler, M. J., Woch, G., and McCall, M. A. (2003). Retinal transplantation-induced recovery of retinotectal visual function in a rodent model of retinitis pigmentosa. *Invest. Ophthalmol. Vis. Sci.* 44(4) :1686-1695.

Sangwan, V. S., Basu, S., Vemuganti, G. K., Sejpal, K., Subramaniam, S. V., Bandyopadhyay, S., et al. (2011). Clinical outcomes of xeno-free autologous cultivated limbal epithelial transplantation: a 10-year study. *Br. J. Ophthalmol.* 95(11): 1525-1529.

Sangwan, V. S., Matalia, H. P., Vemuganti, G. K., Fatima, A., Ifthekar, G., Singh, S., et al. (2006). Clinical outcome of autologous cultivated limbal epithelium transplantation. *Indian. J. Ophthalmol.* 54(1): 29-34.

Sangwan, V. S., Vemuganti, G. K., Iftekhar, G., Bansal, A. K., and Rao, G. N. (2003). Use of autologous cultured limbal and conjunctival epithelium in a patient with severe bilateral ocular surface disease induced by acid injury: a case report of unique application. *Cornea.* 22(5) :478-481.

Schermer, A., Galvin, S., and Sun, T. T. (1986). Differentiation-related expression of a major 64K corneal keratin in vivo and in culture suggests limbal location of corneal epithelial stem cells. *J. Cell Biol.* 103(1):49-62.

Schwartz, S. D., Hubschman, J. P., Heilwell, G., Franco-Cardenas, V., Pan, C. K., Ostrick, R. M., et al. (2012). Embryonic stem cell trials for macular degeneration: a preliminary report. *Lancet.* 379(9817): 713-720.

Secker, G. A., and Daniels, J. T. (2008a). Limbal epithelial stem cells of the cornea. In L. Girard (Ed.), *StemBook* (2010/07/09 ed.). Cambridge (MA) Harvard Stem Cell Institute.

Secker, G. A., and Daniels, J. T. (2008b). Limbal epithelial stem cells of the cornea.

Seiler, M. J., and Aramant, R. B. (2005). Transplantation of neuroblastic progenitor cells as a sheet preserves and restores retinal function. *Semin. Ophthalmol.* 20(1) 31-42.

Seiler, M. J., Aramant, R. B., and Ball, S. L. (1999). Photoreceptor function of retinal transplants implicated by light-dark shift of S-antigen and rod transducin. *Vision Re.,* 39(15): 2589-2596.

Seko, Y., Azuma, N., Kaneda, M., Nakatani, K., Miyagawa, Y., Noshiro, Y., et al. (2012). Derivation of human differential photoreceptor-like cells from the iris by defined combinations of CRX, RX, and NEUROD. *PLoS One.* 7(4) e35611.

Sengupta, N., Caballero, S., Sullivan, S. M., Chang, L. J., Afzal, A., Li Calzi, S., et al. (2009). Regulation of adult hematopoietic stem cells fate for enhanced tissue-specific repair. *Mol. Ther.* 17(9): 1594-1604.

Shortt, A. J., Secker, G. A., Munro, P. M., Khaw, P. T., Tuft, S. J., and Daniels, J. T. (2007). Characterization of the limbal epithelial stem cell niche: novel imaging techniques permit in vivo observation and targeted biopsy of limbal epithelial stem cells. *Stem. Cells.* 25(6): 1402-1409.

Shortt, A. J., Secker, G. A., Rajan, M. S., Meligonis, G., Dart, J. K., Tuft, S. J., et al. (2008). Ex vivo expansion and transplantation of limbal epithelial stem cells. *Ophthalmology.* 115(11): 1989-1997.

Stanga, P. E., Kychenthal, A., Fitzke, F. W., Halfyard, A. S., Chan, R., Bird, A. C., et al. (2002). Retinal pigment epithelium translocation after choroidal neovascular membrane removal in age-related macular degeneration. *Ophthalmology.* 109(8) 1492-1498.

Stepp, M. A., Zhu, L., Sheppard, D., and Cranfill, R. L. (1995). Localized distribution of alpha 9 integrin in the cornea and changes in expression during corneal epithelial cell differentiation. *J. Histochem. Cytochem.* 43(4):353-362.

Stone, L. S. (1965). The Regeneration of the Crystalline Lens. *Invest. Ophthalmol.* 4: 420-432.

Sugino, I. K., Rapista, A., Sun, Q., Wang, J., Nunes, C. F., Cheewatrakoolpong, N., et al. (2011). A method to enhance cell survival on Bruch's membrane in eyes affected by age and age-related macular degeneration. *Invest. Ophthalmol. Vis. Sci.* 52(13): 9598-9609.

Sun, G., Asami, M., Ohta, H., Kosaka, J., and Kosaka, M. (2006). Retinal stem/progenitor properties of iris pigment epithelial cells. *Dev. Biol.* 289(1): 243-252.

Sun, T. T., and Lavker, R. M. (2004). Corneal epithelial stem cells: past, present, and future. *J. Investig. Dermatol. Symp. Proc.* 9(3): 202-207.

Thoft, R. A., and Friend, J. (1983). The X, Y, Z hypothesis of corneal epithelial maintenance. *Invest. Ophthalmol. Vis. Sci.* 24(10): 1442-1443.

Tibbetts, M. D., Samuel, M. A., Chang, T. S., and Ho, A. C. (2012). Stem cell therapy for retinal disease. *Curr. Opin. Ophthalmol.* 23(3) :226-234.

Tropepe, V., Coles, B. L., Chiasson, B. J., Horsford, D. J., Elia, A. J., McInnes, R. R., et al. (2000). Retinal stem cells in the adult mammalian eye. *Science,* 287(5460): 2032-2036.

Tsai, C. L., Wu, P. C., Fini, M. E., and Shi, S. (2011). Identification of multipotent stem/progenitor cells in murine sclera. *Invest. Ophthalmol. Vis. Sci.* 52(8): 5481-5487.

Tseng, S. C. (1989). Concept and application of limbal stem cells. *Eye (Lond)* 3 (Pt 2): 141-157.

Tsonis, P. A., and Del Rio-Tsonis, K. (2004). Lens and retina regeneration: transdifferentiation, stem cells, and clinical applications. *Exp. Eye Res.* 78(2): 161-172.

Tsonis, P. A., and Fuentes, E. J. (2006). Focus on molecules: Pax-6, the eye master. *Exp. Eye Res.* 83(2) :233-234.

Turgeon, P. W., Nauheim, R. C., Roat, M. I., Stopak, S. S., and Thoft, R. A. (1990). Indications for keratoepithelioplasty. *Arch. Ophthalmol.* 108(2): 233-236.

Varghese, V. M., Prasad, T., and Kumary, T. V. (2010). Optimization of culture conditions for an efficient xeno-feeder free limbal cell culture system towards ocular surface regeneration. *Microsc. Res. Tech.* 73(11): 1045-1052.

Vasania, V. S., Prasad, P., Gill, R. K., Mehta, A., Viswanathan, C., Sarang, S., et al. (2011). Molecular and cellular characterization of expanded and cryopreserved human limbal epithelial stem cells reveals unique immunological properties. *Exp. Eye Res.* 92(1): 47-56.

Vastine, D. W., Stewart, W. B., and Schwab, I. R. (1982). Reconstruction of the periocular mucous membrane by autologous conjunctival transplantation. *Ophthalmology.* 89(9): 1072-1081.

Vemuganti, G. K., Fatima, A., Madhira, S. L., Basti, S., and Sangwan, V. S. (2009). Limbal stem cells: application in ocular biomedicine. *Int. Rev. Cell Mol Biol.* 275: 133-181.

Watanabe, K., Nishida, K., Yamato, M., Umemoto, T., Sumide, T., Yamamoto, K., et al. (2004). Human limbal epithelium contains side population cells expressing the ATP-binding cassette transporter ABCG2. *FEBS Lett.* 565(1-3): 6-10.

Wei, Z. G., Cotsarelis, G., Sun, T. T., and Lavker, R. M. (1995). Label-retaining cells are preferentially located in fornical epithelium: implications on conjunctival epithelial homeostasis. *Invest. Ophthalmol. Vis. Sci.* 36(1):236-246.

Wei, Z. G., Lin, T., Sun, T. T., and Lavker, R. M. (1997). Clonal analysis of the in vivo differentiation potential of keratinocytes. *Invest. Ophthalmol. Vis. Sci.* 38(3):753-761.

Wei, Z. G., Wu, R. L., Lavker, R. M., and Sun, T. T. (1993). In vitro growth and differentiation of rabbit bulbar, fornix, and palpebral conjunctival epithelia. Implications on conjunctival epithelial transdifferentiation and stem cells. *Invest. Ophthalmol. Vis. Sci.* 34(5): 1814-1828.

Weisz, J. M., Humayun, M. S., De Juan, E., Jr., Del Cerro, M., Sunness, J. S., Dagnelie, G., et al. (1999). Allogeneic fetal retinal pigment epithelial cell transplant in a patient with geographic atrophy. *Retina.* 19(6):540-545.

West, E. L., Pearson, R. A., Barker, S. E., Luhmann, U. F., Maclaren, R. E., Barber, A. C., et al. (2010). Long-term survival of photoreceptors transplanted into the adult murine neural retina requires immune modulation. *Stem. Cells.* 28(11):1997-2007.

Wirtschafter, J. D., Ketcham, J. M., Weinstock, R. J., Tabesh, T., and McLoon, L. K. (1999). Mucocutaneous junction as the major source of replacement palpebral conjunctival epithelial cells. *Invest. Ophthalmol. Vis. Sci.* 40(13): 3138-3146.

Wohl, S. G., Schmeer, C. W., and Isenmann, S. (2012). Neurogenic potential of stem/progenitor-like cells in the adult mammalian eye. *Prog. Retin. Eye Res.* 31(3): 213-242.

Xu, H., Sta Iglesia, D. D., Kielczewski, J. L., Valenta, D. F., Pease, M. E., Zack, D. J., et al. (2007). Characteristics of progenitor cells derived from adult ciliary body in mouse, rat, and human eyes. *Invest. Ophthalmol. Vis. Sci.* 48(4): 1674-1682.

Yanagi, Y., Inoue, Y., Kawase, Y., Uchida, S., Tamaki, Y., Araie, M., et al. (2006). Properties of growth and molecular profiles of rat progenitor cells from ciliary epithelium. *Exp. Eye Res.* 82(3): 471-478.

Yang, C., Yang, Y., Brennan, L., Bouhassira, E. E., Kantorow, M., and Cvekl, A. (2010). Efficient generation of lens progenitor cells and lentoid bodies from human embryonic stem cells in chemically defined conditions. *FASEB J.* 24(9): 3274-3283.

Yao, Y. F., Inoue, Y., Hara, Y., Kiritoshi, A., Tano, Y., and Ohashi, Y. (1994). Suppression of graft rejection in rat keratoepithelioplasty by anterior chamber inoculation of donor lymphocytes. *Jpn. J. Ophthalmol.* 38(4): 345-352.

Zhang, W., Cveklova, K., Oppermann, B., Kantorow, M., and Cvekl, A. (2001). Quantitation of PAX6 and PAX6(5a) transcript levels in adult human lens, cornea, and monkey retina. *Mol Vis.* 7: 1-5.

Zhou, S., Schuetz, J. D., Bunting, K. D., Colapietro, A. M., Sampath, J., Morris, J. J., et al. (2001). The ABC transporter Bcrp1/ABCG2 is expressed in a wide variety of stem cells and is a molecular determinant of the side-population phenotype. *Nat. Med.* 7(9): 1028-1034.

Index

B

C

D

E

F

G

H

I

J

K

L

M

Q

R

T

U

V

W

Y

Z